Pediatric Bronchoscopy for Clinicians

This book is a quick reference guide and atlas for performing bronchoscopy in pediatric patients. It offers a multidisciplinary approach, incorporating the perspectives of pediatric pulmonology, otolaryngology, anesthesiology, and respiratory therapy by outlining important anatomic and physiologic considerations. It describes the basic and advanced techniques in performing flexible, rigid, and special bronchoscopy maneuvers and approaches. This book enhances the reader's understanding of the critical skill of clinical evaluation and management of the pediatric airway. It is addressed to junior and senior trainees as well as early- and late-career clinicians involved in pediatric bronchoscopy as an on-the-go guide.

KEY FEATURES

- Pays special attention to including widely applicable techniques that can be employed across a variety of domestic and international practical settings, complete with a wealth of accompanying videos and illustrations from real-world experiences that are easy to replicate and reference in practice.
- Promotes a multidisciplinary approach to the evaluation of the upper and lower airways in children with respiratory and aerodigestive pathology as the lines between pediatric pulmonology, otolaryngology, anesthesiology, surgery, critical care, and emergency medicine are blurring, thus providing well-equipped clinicians with a thorough perspective of all disciplines.
- Features bullet-pointed lists for pre-procedure evaluation, with procedural checklists, images, and videos, and serves as a portable, compact, and accessible quick reference guide.

Pediatric Bronchoscopy for Clinicians

Edited by

Don Hayes, Jr., MD, MS, MEd
Professor
Cincinnati Children's Hospital Medical Center
Departments of Pediatrics and Internal Medicine
University of Cincinnati College of Medicine
Cincinnati, Ohio

Kara D. Meister, MD, FAAP, FACS
Clinical Assistant Professor
Aerodigestive & Airway Reconstruction Center
Otolaryngology-Head and Neck Surgery
Division of Pediatric Otolaryngology
Stanford University
Palo Alto, California

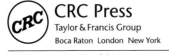

CRC Press
Taylor & Francis Group
Boca Raton London New York

CRC Press is an imprint of the
Taylor & Francis Group, an **informa** business

First edition published 2023
by CRC Press
6000 Broken Sound Parkway NW, Suite 300, Boca Raton, FL 33487-2742

and by CRC Press
4 Park Square, Milton Park, Abingdon, Oxon, OX14 4RN

CRC Press is an imprint of Taylor & Francis Group, LLC

ISBN: 9780367617295 (hbk)
ISBN: 9780367617288 (pbk)
ISBN: 9781003106234 (ebk)

DOI: 10.1201/9781003106234

Typeset in Minion
by Deanta Global Publishing Services, Chennai, India

Access VIDEOS online in Support Materials: www.routledge.com/9780367617288

Dedications

To my wife Keri, my son Hunter, my daughter Kaitlyn, and my grandchildren, whose own accomplishments are a source of great pride for me as they inspire me every day.

D.H.

To my husband Matthew and son Everett who bring love and joy each day.

K.D.M.

Contents

Preface

Pediatric bronchoscopy is an exciting diagnostic tool that has evolved and continues to grow with advancements in technology. Flexible and rigid bronchoscopy allows for a thorough evaluation of the upper and lower airway in children. Most often, these airway evaluations are performed with pediatric pulmonology and pediatric otolaryngology, working as a team to closely examine the entire respiratory tract. With this combined approach expanding rapidly, adequate training is necessary for best results. This book is the first of its kind to fill the training needs of healthcare providers caring for children with airway disorders and lung conditions, at all levels of experience, by providing essential knowledge on all technical aspects of pediatric bronchoscopy.

Understanding clinical indications, basic principles of pediatric bronchoscopy, and commonly encountered diseases or abnormalities is crucial in performing pediatric bronchoscopy. Taking this knowledge and applying it at the bedside with regular practice under the guidance of a mentor can lead to its skillful use. This book is developed by experts who work in pediatric pulmonology and pediatric otolaryngology. Each author is a highly acclaimed clinician and devoted educator focused on teaching others about pediatric bronchoscopy. The goal of this book is to provide insights that will enhance your training and understanding of pediatric bronchoscopy through original and detailed images, videos, and multidisciplinary explanations of the procedures. With a full airway evaluation of children often involving pulmonology and otolaryngology, most of the chapters include a representative of both of these specialties to provide the best insight from a medical and surgical point of view.

The use of a digital platform with a team approach should enhance learning and facilitate the acquisition of skills necessary to perform pediatric bronchoscopy. On behalf of all of the authors, we hope this book facilitates your journey of becoming the best pediatric bronchoscopist you can be.

Don Hayes, Jr., MD, MS, MEd
Kara D. Meister, MD, FAAP, FACS

 Access VIDEOS online in Support Materials: www.routledge.com/9780367617288

Acknowledgments

Our collective team who completed this project would like to acknowledge our mentors, colleagues, trainees, and patients who have been the source of knowledge and inspiration for all of us as educators. We would also like to acknowledge Jose Alejo for his administrative support and efforts with this book.

We would like to thank all the authors who have contributed chapters to this book, and we are grateful to the publishers for their help at every stage of the publication. We would particularly like to thank Himani Dwivedi and Shivangi Pramanik for their tireless efforts and their constant reminders and for putting up with us throughout the editorial process.

Editors

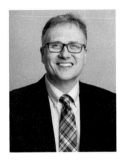

Don Hayes, Jr., MD, MS, MEd, is a pediatric and adult pulmonologist at Cincinnati Children's Hospital Medical Center and the University of Cincinnati Medical Center. He received his medical degree from the University of Kentucky College of Medicine and then completed a combined internal medicine and pediatric residency at East Carolina University Brody School of Medicine. Dr. Hayes then completed a Health Resources and Services Administration (HRSA) Maternal Child Health Bureau–funded fellowship in pediatric pulmonary medicine and a Cystic Fibrosis Foundation–funded fellowship in adult pulmonary disease at the University of Wisconsin School of Medicine and Public Health. During his fellowship, Dr. Hayes concentrated his training in areas of advanced lung disease, lung transplantation, and bronchoscopy. As the Medical Director of the Lung Transplant Program and Co-Director of the Center for End-Stage Lung Failure Program at Cincinnati Children's Hospital Medical Center, Dr. Hayes leads a team of highly recognized clinicians with expertise in a large number of procedures involving bronchoscopy. In addition to using bronchoscopy for clinical reasons, he uses bronchoscopy to study the innate and adaptive immunity of the lung in a variety of chronic pulmonary conditions, including acute and chronic rejection in lung transplant recipients. Dr. Hayes is currently a Professor in the Departments of Pediatrics and Internal Medicine at the University of Cincinnati College of Medicine.

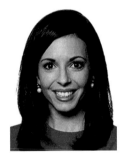

Kara D. Meister, MD, FAAP, FACS, is a Clinical Assistant Professor and Assistant Clinical Chief of Otolaryngology – Head and Neck Surgery Division of Pediatric Otolaryngology at Stanford University. She received her medical degree from the Medical University of South Carolina and then completed her residency in otolaryngology – Head and Neck Surgery at the University of Pittsburgh Medical Center. Dr. Meister completed a fellowship in Pediatric Otolaryngology at Stanford University/Lucile Packard Children's Hospital. Her career is dedicated to the diagnosis, treatment, and investigation of children with complex airway disorders, and she has a special interest in children with congenital heart disease and concurrent airway anomalies. Dr. Meister performs both flexible and rigid bronchoscopy for diagnostic and therapeutic indications across a wide spectrum of pediatric patients. She is a member of the Aerodigestive and Airway Reconstruction Program at Stanford Children's Health. Dr. Meister is a fellow of the American College of Surgeons, the American Academy of Pediatrics, and the American Academy of Otolaryngology – Head & Neck Surgery.

Contributors

Riddhima Agarwal, MS
College of Medicine
The Ohio State University
Columbus, Ohio, USA

Karthik Balakrishnan, MD, MPH, FAAP, FACS
Aerodigestive and Airway Reconstruction
    Center
Department of Otolaryngology
Head and Neck Surgery
Division of Pediatric Otolaryngology
Stanford University
Palo Alto, California, USA

R. Paul Boesch, DO, MS, FAAP
Division of Pediatric Pulmonology
Department of Pediatric and Adolescent
    Medicine
Mayo Clinic Children's Center
Rochester, Minnesota, USA

Gregory Burg, MD
Division of Pulmonary Medicine
Cincinnati Children's Hospital Medical Center
University of Cincinnati College of Medicine
Cincinnati, Ohio, USA

MyMy C. Buu, MD
Division of Pulmonary Medicine
Department of Pediatrics
Stanford University
Palo Alto, California, USA

Tendy Chiang, MD
Center for Regenerative Medicine
Abigail Wexner Research Institute
Department of Pediatric Otolaryngology
Nationwide Children's Hospital
Columbus, Ohio, USA

Antoinette Wannes Daou, MD
Division of Pulmonary Medicine
Department of Pediatrics
Cincinnati Children's Hospital Medical Center
University of Cincinnati College of Medicine
Cincinnati, Ohio, USA

Emily DeBoer, MD
Section of Pulmonary and Sleep Medicine
Department of Pediatrics
University of Colorado Anschutz Medical
    Campus
Aurora, Colorado, USA

Anita Deshpande, MD
Division of Pediatric Otolaryngology
Department of Otolaryngology
Head and Neck Surgery
Cincinnati Children's Hospital Medical Center
University of Cincinnati College of Medicine
Cincinnati, Ohio, USA

Stephen Franklin, DO
Pediatric Pulmonology
Division of Pulmonary Medicine
Children's Hospital of Philadelphia
Philadelphia, Pennsylvania, USA

Catherine K. Hart, MD
Division of Pediatric Otolaryngology
Department of Otolaryngology
Head and Neck Surgery
Cincinnati Children's Hospital Medical Center
University of Cincinnati College of Medicine
Cincinnati, Ohio, USA

Don Hayes, Jr., MD, MS, MEd
Division of Pulmonary Medicine
Department of Pediatrics
Cincinnati Children's Hospital Medical Center
University of Cincinnati College of Medicine
Cincinnati, Ohio, USA

Brandy Johnson MD
Pediatric Pulmonology
Division of Pulmonary Medicine
Children's Hospital of Philadelphia
Philadelphia, Pennsylvania, USA

Maureen Josephson, DO
Pediatric Pulmonology
Division of Pulmonary Medicine
Children's Hospital of Philadelphia
Philadelphia, Pennsylvania, USA

Kimberley R. Kaspy, MD
Division of Pulmonary Medicine
Cincinnati Children's Hospital Medical Center
University of Cincinnati College of Medicine
Cincinnati, Ohio, USA

Katelyn Krivchenia, MD
Division of Pulmonary Medicine
Department of Pediatrics
Nationwide Children's Hospital
The Ohio State University College of Medicine
Columbus, Ohio, USA

Carol Li, MD
Division of Pediatric Otolaryngology
Department of Otolaryngology
Head and Neck Surgery
Cincinnati Children's Hospital Medical Center
University of Cincinnati College of Medicine
Cincinnati, Ohio, USA

Meredith Merz Lind, MD
Department of Pediatric Otolaryngology
Nationwide Children's Hospital
Department of Otolaryngology
The Ohio State University College of Medicine
Columbus, Ohio, USA

Kara D. Meister, MD, FAAP, FACS
Aerodigestive and Airway Reconstruction
    Center
Department of Otolaryngology
Head and Neck Surgery
Division of Pediatric Otolaryngology
Stanford University
Palo Alto, California, USA

Melissa Brooks Peterson, MD
Department of Anesthesiology
University of Colorado School of Medicine
University of Colorado Anschutz Medical
    Campus
Aurora, Colorado, USA

Pelton Phinizy, MD
Center for Pediatric Airway Disorders
Division of Pulmonary and Sleep Medicine
Perelman School of Medicine at The University
    of Pennsylvania
Philadelphia, Pennsylvania, USA

Jeremy D. Prager, MD
Department of Otolaryngology
Head and Neck Surgery
University of Colorado School of Medicine
Children's Hospital Colorado
Aurora, Colorado, USA

Joshua Shannon, BSRT, RRT
Division of Pulmonary Medicine
Cincinnati Children's Hospital Medical Center
Cincinnati, Ohio, USA

Douglas R. Sidell, MD, FAAP, FACS
Aerodigestive and Airway Reconstruction
    Center
Department of Otolaryngology
Head and Neck Surgery
Division of Pediatric Otolaryngology
Stanford University
Palo Alto, California, USA

Cherie A. Torres-Silva, MD, MPH, MEd
Division of Pulmonary Medicine
Department of Pediatrics
Cincinnati Children's Hospital Medical Center
University of Cincinnati College of Medicine
Cincinnati, Ohio, USA

Christopher Towe, MD
Division of Pulmonary Medicine
Department of Pediatrics
Cincinnati Children's Hospital Medical Center
University of Cincinnati College of Medicine
Cincinnati, Ohio, USA

Carolyn Wallace, MHA, RRT-NPS
Division of Pulmonary Medicine
Cincinnati Children's Hospital Medical Center
Cincinnati, Ohio, USA

Sara M. Zak, MD
Division of Pulmonary Medicine
Department of Pediatrics
Cincinnati Children's Hospital Medical Center
University of Cincinnati College of Medicine
Cincinnati, Ohio, USA

Clinical indications for bronchoscopy

KATELYN KRIVCHENIA AND MEREDITH MERZ LIND

INTRODUCTION

Bronchoscopy in children offers clinicians the ability to directly interact with the airway for the purposes of diagnosis and treatment. Both rigid and flexible bronchoscopes are utilized to evaluate upper and lower airway anatomy, assess airway dynamics, collect clinical samples, and administer therapeutic interventions. There are many differences between rigid and flexible bronchoscopes, each tool having benefits and drawbacks depending on the patient, the intended task, and the clinical scenario. Often, these tools work best when used in tandem to better understand airway and lung pathology.

In this chapter, we discuss the advantages bronchoscopy may have over clinical assessment and imaging studies in a child. We review the clinical applications of rigid and flexible bronchoscopy and discuss the benefits and limitations of each so that the reader can better appreciate their appropriate use. Finally, we will review a patient case, demonstrating the way these approaches can be used together clinically.

ADVANTAGES OF BRONCHOSCOPY OVER CLINICAL ASSESSMENT AND CHEST RADIOGRAPHY

Although the foundation of medical practice and clinical decision making will always be a comprehensive history and physical examination, patient factors may complicate clinical assessment, especially in the pediatric population. Difficulty in obtaining an appropriate history and poor cooperation during physical examination are common issues in assessing a young child. Additionally, symptoms such as stridor or wheezing can be the result of an obstruction in multiple locations in the airway and, even in the case of a cooperative child allowing a comprehensive examination, the acoustics of the pediatric chest may make it difficult to localize pathology. Given this, additional procedures are often required in the pediatric patient to gather information and appropriately diagnose pathology.

The field of diagnostic imaging is rapidly expanding, with numerous new techniques and software reconstructions in computed tomography (CT) and magnetic resonance imaging (MRI). These allow for 3-D reconstruction of the lungs and airways to aid in clinical decision making. Techniques such as volumetric imaging of the airway during free breathing ("4-D CT") and multidetector CT ("virtual bronchoscopy") have proven accurate in diagnosing tracheobronchomalacia and foreign bodies in airways.[1–3] Despite these advances, imaging techniques cannot replace bronchoscopy in its unique ability to directly visualize and accurately measure airway pathology or dynamic change. For patients who are critically ill and unable to be transported for imaging procedures, bronchoscopy may offer a bedside alternative for evaluation. Additionally, there is no radiographic substitute for the diagnostic and therapeutic interventions which both rigid and flexible bronchoscopy provide.

The decision to pursue imaging procedures *versus* bronchoscopic intervention will ultimately need to be determined for each individual patient, while considering a multitude of patient and system factors. Patient condition, index of suspicion for particular clinical diagnoses that might require urgent operative intervention, previous radiation exposure or anesthetic complications, availability of imaging modalities and well-trained clinicians, and shared decision making with families, among other factors, will impact the decision to pursue one modality or the other. In some cases, both imaging and bronchoscopy will be essential in determining diagnosis or treatment.

CLINICAL APPLICATIONS OF RIGID BRONCHOSCOPY

EVALUATE AIRWAY ANATOMY

The practice of rigid bronchoscopy involves the use of several specialized instruments (Figure 1.1) that can be used in a variety of configurations, depending on the patient's particular anatomy, as well as on the goals of the procedure and the intervention. Visualization of the airway in rigid bronchoscopy was traditionally performed *via* a rigid ventilating bronchoscope (Figure 1.1C) and the naked eye but now typically involves the use of a rigid fiber-optic telescope that contains a series of high-resolution glass rod lenses (Figure 1.1A and E). This type of telescope provides superior optical quality over flexible fiber-optic scopes, as well as the ability to take still photographs and video. Under sedation and using a rigid laryngoscope and either an unsheathed optical telescope or telescope seated in a rigid ventilating bronchoscope, the oral, pharyngeal, and laryngeal structures can be visualized at high resolution on a video screen. The telescope or bronchoscope can then be passed into the subglottic airway, where the subglottis, trachea, and mainstem bronchi can be visualized. Typically, the first or second divisions of the bronchi can be visualized, but smaller airways may not be accessed with rigid equipment.

Rigid laryngoscopy and bronchoscopy require collaboration between the endoscopist and the anesthesiologist to determine the best anesthetic technique for a particular patient and procedure. Ideally, the patient will be sedated but allowed to breathe spontaneously, which allows ample time to evaluate the airways. This plane of anesthesia may be difficult to maintain in certain patients, and time for evaluation may be limited or require the use of a ventilating bronchoscope, allowing for delivery of positive pressure ventilation when placed into the lower airway. Additionally, other patient factors, including mouth-opening and craniofacial, neck, and spine anatomy, may make accessing the airway with a rigid bronchoscope difficult or even impossible. In these cases, flexible bronchoscopy may be more appropriate to obtain a comprehensive view of the airway.

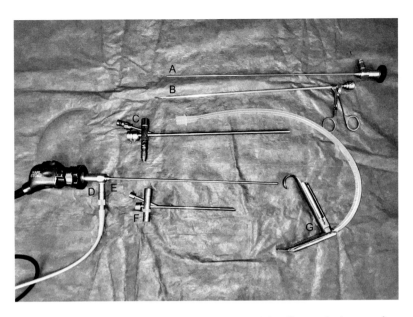

Figure 1.1 Rigid laryngoscopy and bronchoscopy equipment. (A) Small optical telescope for use with optical forceps, (B) optical coin-grasping forceps, (C) rigid ventilating bronchoscope, (D) camera and light cord, (E) 4-mm optical telescope for use with a rigid bronchoscope, (F) small rigid bronchoscope, and (G) Parson's laryngoscope with an adapter for the mechanical ventilator.

Assess airway dynamics

Assessment of airway dynamics can be performed in several ways and often benefits from visualization with multiple techniques. In most cases, evaluation of the dynamics of the upper airway, including the nose, nasopharynx, oropharynx, and supraglottis/glottis is best performed with a flexible endoscope in an awake patient (Video 1.1). However, patient anatomy or cooperation may make the evaluation of these structures difficult, and a sedated procedure may be required. In this case, rigid laryngoscopy and visualization with a fiber-optic telescope in a sedated but spontaneously breathing patient can be an excellent alternative for visualization of the supraglottic and glottic structures (Video 1.2), with the added ability to evaluate the dynamics of the subglottic and tracheal airway. The presence of the laryngoscope may alter the position and anatomy of these structures, however, and this should be considered. Additionally, the mobility of the vocal folds should be determined in an awake patient whenever possible, as anesthesia may affect the mobility and responsiveness of the glottis.

Video 1.1 Laryngomalacia viewed *via* flexible nasopharyngoscopy in an awake infant.

Video 1.2 Laryngomalacia viewed *via* rigid laryngoscope in an anesthetized infant.

In most patients, the dynamic structure of the trachea can be well assessed with a rigid fiber-optic telescope, which, if appropriately sized, does not alter the position or structure of the tracheal airway. The presence, location, and severity of tracheomalacia can be determined and documented, as well as the degree and configuration of external compression and pulsatility in these areas. Similarly, proximal bronchomalacia can be evaluated with a rigid telescope or bronchoscope. Finally, the use of a rigid ventilating bronchoscope allows for the delivery of titrated positive pressure. This may allow for visualization and localization of a

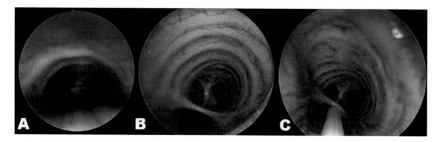

Figure 1.2 Tracheoesophageal fistula in distal trachea (A) without positive pressure, (B) with positive pressure, and (C) with Fogarty catheter in place. See rigid bronchoscopy Video 1.1.

tracheoesophageal fistula or may be of therapeutic benefit to determine appropriate positive pressure to overcome severe tracheomalacia in ventilator-dependent patients (**Figure 1.2, Video 1.3**).

Video 1.3 Severe vascular compression of the left mainstem bronchus, viewed by flexible bronchoscopy.

OBTAIN CLINICAL SAMPLES

In addition to the superior optical quality of rigid bronchoscopes, their benefit, especially in the pediatric patient, is the ability to instrument the airway for diagnosis and treatment. The small size of pediatric flexible bronchoscopes limits the working channel size and functionality. Given this, many biopsies and clinical samples are more easily obtained using rigid instrumentation. Lesions of the supraglottic, glottic, and subglottic airway can be biopsied using a rigid laryngoscope placed into suspension with the use of an operating microscope or optical telescope. A mucosal-covered lesion in the subglottis of a young infant might be concerning for a subglottic hemangioma (**Figure 1.3**). Tissue biopsy can confirm this diagnosis, so that medical therapy with propranolol can be initiated.

Lower airway lesions can likewise be sampled using a ventilating bronchoscope, with optical forceps inserted through the scope or inserted directly into the airway through the laryngoscope. Diagnosis of primary ciliary dyskinesia often requires cilia biopsy with electron microscopy evaluation, and distal tracheal mucosal biopsies are often desired for this purpose. Purulent or otherwise abnormal secretions can be directly

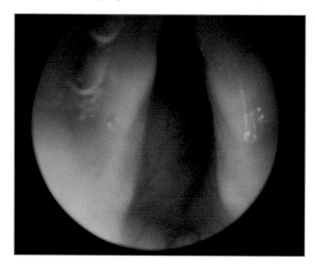

Figure 1.3 Subglottic hemangioma in the most common position, namely left posterior subglottis.

visualized with an optical telescope and suctioned for culture *via* a flexible suction catheter deployed through a rigid bronchoscope. Likewise, saline can be delivered *via* a suction catheter and collected for bronchoalveolar lavage (BAL) if a particular situation does not allow for concurrent flexible bronchoscopy for this purpose.

THERAPEUTIC INTERVENTION

The therapeutic functions that the rigid bronchoscope and its associated accessories can perform may be too numerous to list. One benefit that rigid bronchoscopy has over imaging and other procedures is the ability to diagnose and concurrently treat many airway pathologies. Based on patient history, symptoms, and condition, the appropriate instruments should be available and assembled prior to initiation of the procedure, although the array of procedures that can be performed with appropriate instruments is broad and, in many cases, can be adjusted intraoperatively without a major change in equipment, patient preparation, or anesthetic plan.

Supraglottic and glottic pathology can be addressed using a rigid laryngoscope placed into suspension, with the use of either an operating microscope and bi-manual instrumentation or an optical telescope and one-handed instrumentation. Supraglottoplasty can be performed to treat severe laryngomalacia (**Figure 1.4, Video 1.2** and **Video 1.3**). Vallecular and laryngeal cysts (**Figure 1.5**) can be excised to relieve airway obstruction. Vocal fold lesions, such as cysts, nodules, or papillomas (**Figure 1.6**), can be excised using microscopic instruments, powered instrumentation, or a laser. Certain glottic webs (**Figure 1.7**) can be divided and stents can be placed endoscopically to avoid opening the airway and laryngofissure.

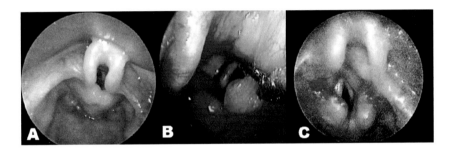

Figure 1.4 Laryngomalacia viewed by rigid laryngoscope (A) prior to supraglottoplasty, (B) during supraglottoplasty after incision of the left aryepiglottic fold, and (C) supraglottoplasty after incision of the bilateral aryepiglottic folds.

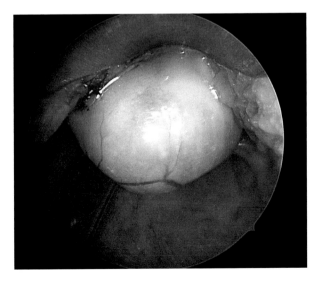

Figure 1.5 Vallecular cyst with endotracheal tube in place.

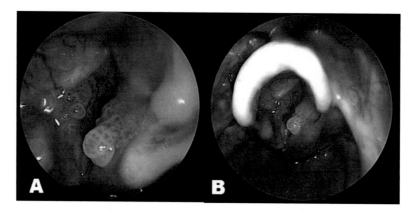

Figure 1.6 Recurrent respiratory papillomatosis involving the glottic (A) and supraglottic (B) structures.

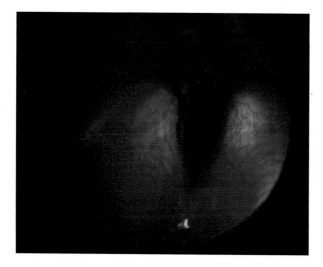

Figure 1.7 Congenital anterior glottic web.

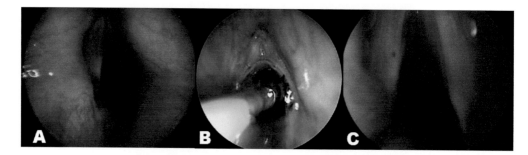

Figure 1.8 Grade 3 subglottic stenosis (A) before dilation, (B) during balloon dilation, and (C) after dilation.

Both congenital and acquired lesions can be seen in the subglottis. When they occur, complications from intubation are most often seen in this portion of the airway. Granulomas and cysts may form here because of endotracheal tube placement and can be excised using sharp or powered instrumentation. Early acquired subglottic stenosis can be dilated with a balloon to prevent permanent scarring that would require open-airway surgery to correct (**Figure 1.8**). More mature stenosis can be addressed with laser division followed by dilatation. Therapeutic injections with glucosteroid or other medications can also be performed endoscopically.

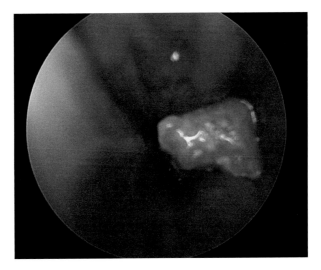

Figure 1.9 Obstructing tracheal granuloma at the superior tracheostoma.

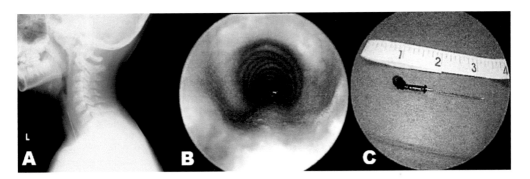

Figure 1.10 (A) Lateral neck X-ray, showing a foreign body in the trachea. (B) Tracheal foreign body prior to removal. (C) Homemade "blow dart" after removal from airway.

Using a rigid ventilating bronchoscope or optical instruments, lesions in the trachea can be excised endoscopically. Patients with tracheostomy may develop intraluminal stomal granulomas that can cause obstruction (Figure 1.9). These can be removed *via* bronchoscopy. Other lesions can be excised for biopsy and relief of symptoms. Airway casts and mucus plugs that are too large or tenacious to be removed with a flexible bronchoscope can be removed using larger suction or optical instruments *via* a rigid bronchoscope.

Foreign body aspiration into the airway can be life-threatening and may not be witnessed or suspected, especially in a young child. History, physical examination, or imaging studies may raise concern for possible aspirated foreign objects, although the gold standard for diagnosis of this condition is with rigid bronchoscopy, and a high index of suspicion is essential so that diagnosis is not missed. In addition to diagnosis, therapeutic intervention can be immediately performed with rigid bronchoscopic equipment (Figure 1.10). Foreign bodies can become lodged at any point in the airway, including in the pharynx, glottis, trachea, or, most commonly, the bronchi (Figure 1.11). Various equipment can be used to access and remove foreign objects located at any point in the airway down to the first or second bronchial divisions. Endoscopists should be intimately familiar with their equipment and its function in order to care for these patients efficiently and safely. More distal objects might be accessed with flexible bronchoscopy, and, in very rare cases, open surgery may be required to remove a foreign body.

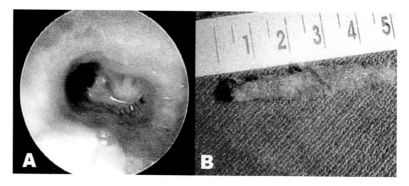

Figure 1.11 Organic foreign body (grass) in the right mainstem bronchus (A) and after removal (B).

CLINICAL APPLICATIONS OF FLEXIBLE BRONCHOSCOPY

EVALUATE AIRWAY ANATOMY

The size and flexibility of the scopes used for flexible bronchoscopy allow the practitioner to gain access to smaller and more distant airways than is possible with the rigid scope. The airway can be entered *via* the nasal passageways for an evaluation of nasopharyngeal and laryngeal structures without the impact of the positioning needed for the rigid bronchoscope. The subglottic space and upper trachea are visualized when entering *via* the nasal passageways or through a laryngeal mask airway (LMA). Finally, the distal trachea, bilateral mainstem bronchi, or branching segments/subsegments can be visually explored regardless of whether the airway was entered through the nose, LMA, endotracheal tube (ETT), or tracheostomy tube. Depending on the size of the scope and the child, several branching subsegments may be accessible.

During the procedure, the clinician will visualize airway structures to assess for narrowing from intrinsic or external causes, such as bronchial stenosis or airway compression (from vascular structures, lymph nodes, masses, etc.), respectively. The airway mucosa is evaluated for abnormalities suggesting chronic or acute inflammation (Figure 1.12), in addition to changes indicating vascular (Figure 1.13) or infectious abnormalities. Clinicians use the presence, volume, and consistency of secretions in various locations to help with diagnostic or therapeutic medical interventions. Finally, the identification of an intraluminal foreign

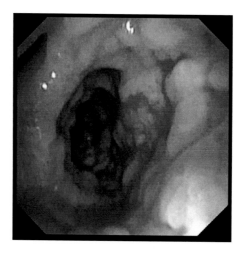

Figure 1.12 Acutely inflamed airway mucosa in patient with non-cystic fibrosis bronchiectasis.

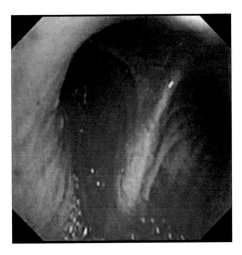

Figure 1.13 Acute airway bleeding in a patient with polyangiitis with granulomatosis.

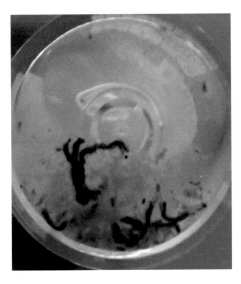

Figure 1.14 Airway cast of aspirated feculent material from lavage of intubated ICU patient.

body, mucus plug, airway cast (**Figure 1.14**), or endobronchial mass can reveal the cause of initial presenting symptoms or radiographic abnormalities.

ASSESS AIRWAY DYNAMICS

The mechanics of the flexible scope allow for the assessment of upper and lower airway dynamics while avoiding the airway tension/positioning required for rigid bronchoscopy, which could potentially alter findings of airway malacia or narrowing. The ideal assessment of airway dynamics would involve a nasopharyngeal approach in a spontaneously breathing child so that the pharyngeal, laryngeal, tracheal, and bronchial dynamics can be assessed in a setting most closely mimicking the child's sleeping physiology. Drug-induced sleep endoscopy (DISE) is the practice of performing nasolaryngoscopy while a child is in drug-simulated sleep, to assess areas of obstruction in children with obstructive sleep apnea. This approach allows the practitioner to assess for significant airway obstruction in each anatomic structure with easy breathing. The visualization of a cough or agitation during the procedure can also impart valuable knowledge relating to the child's airway dynamics under stress. Additionally, airway narrowing can be further described as pulsatile or static,

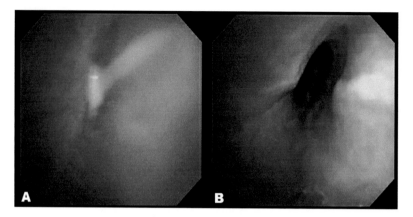

Figure 1.15 Compression of the left mainstem bronchus (A) before and (B) after surgical aortopexy.

aiding in differentiation between vascular and non-vascular causes of compression (**Video 1.3**). Similar to the use of rigid bronchoscopy in tracheomalacia, the flexible bronchoscope can be utilized to help determine the benefit of intervention with increased ventilatory pressures or the impact of other intra-operative procedures, such as stenting of the pulmonary artery or aortopexy (**Figure 1.15**) on the more distal airways.

Depending on the clinical scenario and typical institutional practice, the bronchoscopist may need to enter the subglottic airway through an LMA or ETT. An assessment of dynamic airway change is still possible in this setting, although the practitioner must account for the limitations of these approaches as they interpret the findings. An LMA will alter laryngeal positioning and appearance, whereas the ETT will bypass the subglottic space and stent the proximal trachea open in a way that may prevent adequate assessment of tracheomalacia. Additionally, when an ETT is used to enter the airway, it must be noted that the flexible bronchoscope takes up a significant amount of space in the tube, particularly in infants and small children. This creates an element of positive end-expiratory pressure (PEEP) that is difficult to measure and may effectively mask lower airway malacia that would otherwise be visualized.

OBTAIN CLINICAL SAMPLES

The information obtained from BAL can be vital to the clinician as a diagnostic tool, offering a window into processes at the alveolar level. Cytological studies on the BAL fluid may alert the provider to the presence and nature of cellular inflammation, evidence of alveolar hemorrhage or proteinosis, and characteristics of infectious pathogens. BAL fluid can be further analyzed for microbial culture and infectious studies. Bronchial brushings can provide information on cellular make-up and the pathology of the airway mucosa.

In the correct clinical setting, endobronchial and transbronchial biopsies can be performed in a way that targets abnormal airway or lung tissue without the risk of more invasive surgical procedures. The utility of this is more restricted in the pediatric population due to the size limitations of the bronchoscope. More advanced and specialized bronchoscopic procedures continue to be developed for ongoing improvement of diagnostic yield.

THERAPEUTIC INTERVENTION

The therapeutic utility of a flexible bronchoscope mostly revolves around its ability to suction, lavage, and instill medication in the more distal airways inaccessible to the rigid bronchoscope. The skilled clinician can clear various types and consistencies of secretions, mucus plugs, and airway casts (**Figure 1.16**) to improve ventilation and/or oxygenation. Serial lavages of normal saline can assist in clearing even more distal airways and can be utilized by experienced hands to treat pulmonary alveolar proteinosis.

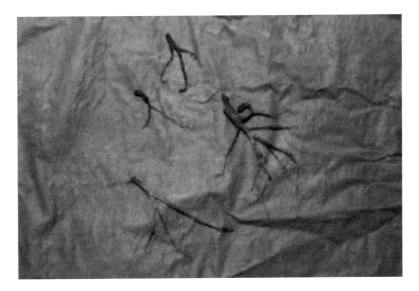

Figure 1.16 Multiple airway casts removed in patient with plastic bronchitis.

In the intensive care setting, bronchoscopy may be utilized to help locally instill various medications to target airway bleeding, recurrent mucus plugging, or persistent air leaks as patient size and clinical scenarios allow.

CASE PRESENTATION

- A teenage male with a history of Chiari type I malformation, prior tracheoesophageal fistula status post-repair, tracheobronchomalacia, unrepaired laryngeal cleft, dysphagia, and tracheostomy dependence presents for evaluation and repair of his laryngeal cleft.
- Non-contrast CT of the neck and chest shows some thinning of mucosa between the trachea and the esophagus without definite communication (Figure 1.17).

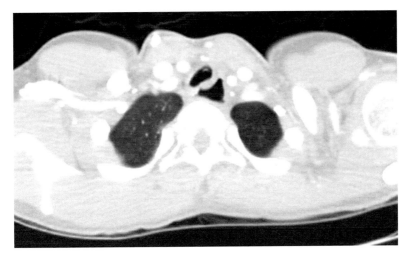

Figure 1.17 Axial CT imaging showing some thinning of mucosa between the trachea and the esophagus, without definite communication.

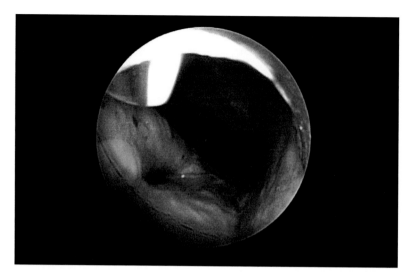

Figure 1.18 Large tracheoesophageal fistula on posterior tracheal wall.

- Airway evaluation is arranged by direct laryngoscopy, rigid bronchoscopy, and flexible bronchoscopy with BAL. These are coordinated with an esophagogastroduodenoscopy ("Triple Endoscopy").
- Laryngoscopy reveals a deep Type 3 laryngeal cleft without stenosis.
- Rigid bronchoscopy shows a well-positioned tracheostoma. Close evaluation of the posterior tracheal wall reveals a large tracheoesophageal fistula just below the tracheostoma (Figure 1.18, Video 1.4).
- Subsequent flexible bronchoscopy reveals findings of chronic mucosal inflammation. BAL reveals normal cytology with predominant mono/macrophages, with few neutrophils and no microbial growth from cultures.
- Endoscopy demonstrates friable esophageal mucosa with eosinophilic inflammation on biopsy.
- The patient tolerates the above procedures well, with plans for surgical repair of his tracheoesophageal fistula and laryngeal cleft.

Video 1.4 Tracheoesophageal fistula in the distal trachea during rigid bronchoscopy.

CONCLUSION

Both rigid and flexible bronchoscopy have many clinical applications in the diagnosis and treatment of airway conditions in children. Each procedure has advantages and drawbacks over the other (Table 1.1), and the use of one or both procedures should be considered in light of the suspected pathology and the goals of treatment in each individual patient. Certain clinical conditions may benefit from the use of concurrent flexible and rigid bronchoscopic procedures.

TIPS FOR CLINICAL PRACTICE

- Prior to pursuing bronchoscopy, an appropriate history and physical examination should be obtained, and available imaging studies should be reviewed.

- The clinical status, comorbid medical conditions, suspected diagnosis, and goals of treatment for each patient should be considered when deciding on the most appropriate bronchoscopic procedure. Often a combination of approaches, with both rigid and flexible bronchoscopes, may be indicated.
- Repeated airway evaluations may be required, depending on the underlying pathology.

Table 1.1 Comparison of flexible and rigid pediatric bronchoscopy

	Rigid bronchoscopy	Flexible bronchoscopy
Advantages	**Airway anatomy** • Superior optical quality **Airway dynamics** • Evaluation of the upper and lower airway structures during spontaneous ventilation. • With a ventilating bronchoscope, can determine the amount of pressure needed to overcome airway malacia • Visualization and instrumentation of an occult tracheoesophageal fistula can be performed **Obtain clinical samples** • Easy to obtain tissue biopsies using optical forceps • Direct suctioning of secretions **Therapeutic intervention** • Diagnosis and treatment of many conditions during the same procedure • Multitude of associated instruments to perform many intra-airway procedures • Innumerable functions including biopsy, foreign body removal, excision of masses/lesions, airway dilation, treatment of airway stenosis, and more	**Airway anatomy** • Visualization of more distal airways • Not typically patient position dependent, so can be used in patients with anatomic constraints • Can be performed via nasal passage, LMA, or endotracheal/tracheostomy tube **Airway dynamics** • Upper airway anatomy is best viewed in an awake patient with a flexible scope • Upper airway endoscopy during simulated sleep can be performed • Less likely to deform or stent the airway during dynamic evaluation **Obtain clinical samples** • Better option is to obtain clinical samples from the distal airways • Flexible scope can be "wedged" into the airway to administer and collect BAL fluid **Therapeutic intervention** • Suctioning and clearance of secretions or mucus plugs from the small/distal airways • Targeted instillation of medications
Drawbacks	**Airway anatomy** • Cannot access/visualize smaller airways • Requires collaboration with anesthesiologist for concurrent patient ventilation • Patient anatomy may make access difficult **Airway dynamics** • Rigid scopes may alter airway anatomy **Obtain clinical samples** • Difficult to "wedge" bronchoscope for BAL collection **Therapeutic intervention** • Difficult to reach right upper lobe or distal bronchi in some patients	**Airway anatomy** • Poorer optical quality **Airway dynamics** • When using LMA or endotracheal tube, dynamics may be altered • Bronchoscope in ETT contributes to PEEP during the procedure and may alter the airway assessment **Obtain clinical samples** • More difficult to obtain biopsies in younger patients due to the small size of the scope and instruments **Therapeutic intervention** • Limited use due to small size of scope and instruments

REFERENCES

1. Lee KS, Sun MRM, Ernst A, et al. Comparison of dynamic expiratory CT with bronchoscopy for diagnosing airway malacia: a pilot evaluation. *Chest*. 2007 Mar;131(3):758–764.
2. Andronikou S, Chopra M, Langton-Hewer S, et al. Technique, pitfalls, quality, radiation dose and findings of dynamic 4-dimensional computed tomography for airway imaging in infants and children. *Pediatr Radiol*. 2019 May;49(5):678–686.
3. Behera G, Tripathy N, Maru YK, et al. Role of virtual bronchoscopy in children with a vegetable foreign body in the tracheobronchial tree. *J Laryngol Otol*. 2014 Dec;128(12):1078–1083.

2

Basics of flexible bronchoscopy and equipment

ANTOINETTE WANNES DAOU, CAROLYN WALLACE,
JOSHUA SHANNON, AND CHERIE A. TORRES-SILVA

DOI: 10.1201/9781003106234-2

INTRODUCTION

WHAT IS FLEXIBLE BRONCHOSCOPY?

Flexible bronchoscopy is an endoscopic technique for visualization of the inside of the airways for diagnostic and therapeutic purposes. A flexible, fiber-optic bronchoscope is inserted into the airways, through the nose, mouth, or artificial airway. Flexible bronchoscopy is performed with the purpose of identification and characterization of anatomical or dynamic abnormalities and/or obstructions, congenital anomalies, infection, inflammation, or endobronchial lesions. In addition, bronchoscopy is performed as a therapeutic procedure to remove secretions, mucus plugs, casts, blood clots, and foreign bodies, as well as to perform interventional diagnostic or therapeutic procedures including laser cauterization, cryoablation, balloon dilatation, or biopsies.[1]

Common indications for bronchoscopic evaluation include chronic respiratory symptoms, recurrent lower respiratory infections, hemoptysis, obstructive sleep apnea, and mucus clearance impairment (Table 2.1).[2,3]

ABOUT THE INSTRUMENTS: FLEXIBLE *VERSUS* RIGID BRONCHOSCOPES

FLEXIBLE BRONCHOSCOPES

Flexible fiber-optic bronchoscopes were introduced in the early 1970s. The flexible bronchoscope allows for evaluation of the anatomy and dynamics of the upper and lower airways. These instruments, except for the 2.2-mm neonatal-size bronchoscope, have a suction/working channel which ranges in diameter from 1.2 to 2.8 mm. The working channel allows for suctioning of secretions or bronchoalveolar lavage sample collection, instillation of fluid, insufflation of oxygen, and passage of small instruments, such as cytology brushes, laser probes, cryoprobes, and biopsy forceps.[4]

Table 2.1 What are indications of flexible bronchoscopy?

Indications	
Diagnostic	**Need for information within the lungs or airways:** • Upper airway obstruction • Chronic cough • Lower airway cultures needed • Abnormal imaging • Localization of bleeding • Severe persistent asthma, difficult to treat • Extubation failure • Biopsies – transbronchial, endobronchial.
Therapeutic	**Need to relieve obstruction in the airways:** • Improve atelectasis due to mucus plugging • Removal of foreign body
Intubation assistance	• Elective, nasotracheal intubation • Difficult view • Spinal issues

ADVANTAGES OF FLEXIBLE BRONCHOSCOPY OVER RIGID BRONCHOSCOPY

Flexible bronchoscopy has the capacity to:

- Evaluate airways in patients for whom passage of the rigid bronchoscope is problematic (mandibular hypoplasia, cervical or temporomandibular ankyloses, severe kyphoscoliosis, and patients with an unstable cervical spine)
- Evaluate airway dynamics without causing distortion of the anatomy which would be affected by the rigid bronchoscope.
- Evaluate lower airways through an established artificial airway.
- Access and visualize the bronchi of the lung apices, as well as more peripheral smaller airways.[4,5]

ADVANTAGES OF PERFORMING A COMBINED AIRWAY EVALUATION

Performing a combined airway evaluation, including flexible and rigid bronchoscopy, allows for a complete anatomic and dynamic assessment of the entire airway.[1,6]

- Rigid bronchoscopy will provide a detailed evaluation of the anatomical structure of the larynx and central airways.
- Flexible bronchoscopy will give detailed evaluation of the anatomical structure of the supraglottic area and the lower airways beyond the carina, will evaluate the dynamics of the upper and lower airways, and will collect bronchoalveolar lavage (BAL) to evaluate for infection, inflammation, and/or potential markers of ongoing aspiration.

EQUIPMENT

THE MINIMUM EQUIPMENT WE RECOMMEND FOR A BRONCHOSCOPY PROGRAM

- 2 × 2.8 mm/3.1 mm flexible bronchoscopes (pediatric bronchoscopes)
- 1 × 4.2 mm bronchoscope or equivalent with a 2.0-mm suction channel (adult bronchoscope)
- 1 × light source
- 1 × video processor
- 1 × video monitor
- 1 × video recording system

The light source, video processor, video monitor, and video recording system can be mounted in the operating room (OR) suite or to a portable cart (Figures 2.1 and 2.2). Procedures should be recorded, and snapshot images of findings should be taken to show the patient and family what was seen during the procedure.

BRONCHOSCOPY SUPPLY ITEMS

For the procedure include (equipment and quantity may vary depending on patient and hospital setting) (Figure 2.3):[3,7]

- 10 mL slip-tip syringes (fill with saline for bronchoalveolar lavage [BAL])
- Suction tubing
- Suction catheter kit
- Specimen trap (for BAL specimen collection)
- Bottle of sodium chloride (for BAL and mucus clearance)
- Oxygen tubing (for airway insufflation to relieve obstruction)

2% lidocaine (local anesthesia for the vocal cords and carina)
- Oxymetazoline (to dilate nasal passage) as indicated

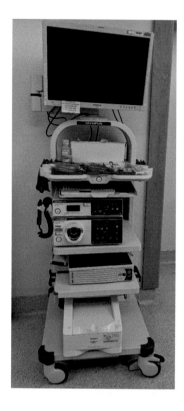

Figure 2.1 Bronchoscopy cart.

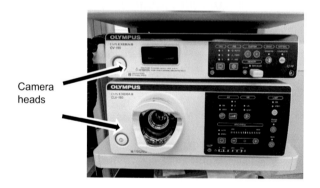

Figure 2.2 Light source. Black arrows indicate camera heads.

- Suction valve for scope
- Biopsy valve for scope
- Ventilator bronchoscope elbow (connects to ventilator, for ventilation during procedure)
- Specimen bags (for transport of clinical samples to Pathology and Microbiology)

COMPONENTS OF THE FLEXIBLE BRONCHOSCOPE (FIGURES 2.4, 2.5, AND 2.6)

- *Light source*: Provides light for image. When cleaning the bronchoscope, the light source must have a gas cap tightly on; if not, the entire bronchoscope and its electrical system can become flooded and damaged during the cleaning process.
- *Suction valve*: Allows for suctioning of secretions and insufflation of oxygen.

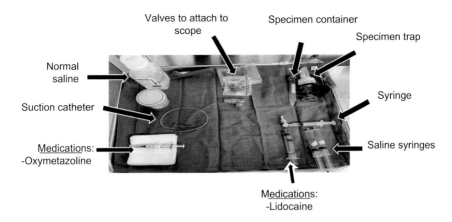

Figure 2.3 Setup before flexible bronchoscopy.

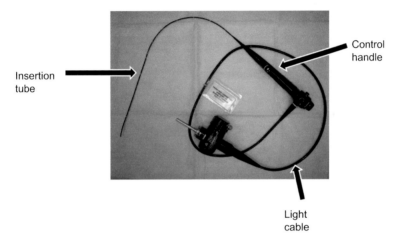

Figure 2.4 Components of flexible bronchoscope.

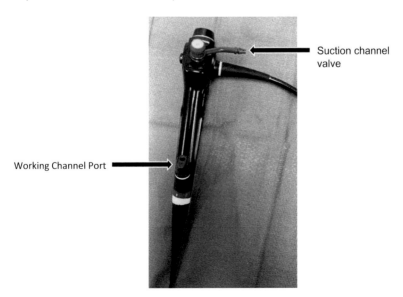

Figure 2.5 Suction channel and working port.

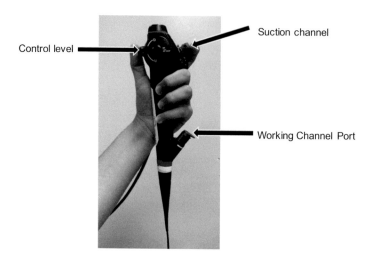

Figure 2.6 Control handle.

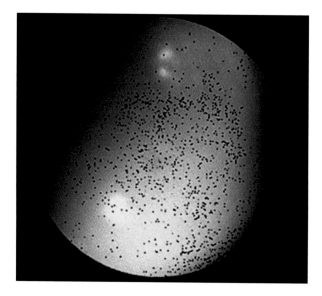

Figure 2.7 Damage of fiber-optic fibers.

- *Working channel port*: Used to provide medication, saline, and to advance therapeutic tools.
- *Control lever*: Controls the tip by two wires extending laterally from the handle to the tip in the insertion cord.
- *Insertion cord*: Contains fiber-optic bundle for light and image transmission. Cord contains thousands of very delicate fibers. If fibers are broken, image is compromised (**Figure 2.7**).[7,8]

BASICS OF HANDLING A FLEXIBLE BRONCHOSCOPE

Flexible bronchoscopes are expensive and fragile instruments. These instruments are designed to be waterproof, so that a leak through the skin or the suction channel can cause damage to the instrument and lead to nosocomial infections. Internal damage to the bronchoscope can be caused by incorrectly passing therapeutic tools through the working channel (i.e., biopsy forceps). Damage to the external covering of the bronchoscope can be caused by direct abrasion to the cover (e.g., passage through an artificial airway). When performing flexible bronchoscopy through an endotracheal tube, it is imperative to use a bite block[8,9] to protect the instrument from the patient biting the shaft, which can permanently damage the fiber optics, as shown by the presence of multiple black dots in the video image (Figure 2.7).

PREPARATION FOR A FLEXIBLE BRONCHOSCOPY

Any bronchoscopic procedure should be safe and comfortable for the patient. Sedation of patients, either conscious sedation or general anesthesia, is strongly recommended to decrease the possibility of bodily or psychological harm. Sedation and monitoring during the procedure should be done by a trained and credentialed provider. The advantage of utilizing "anesthesia" rather than "sedation" is the use of agents like intravenous (IV) propofol and inhaled sevoflurane, which have a very rapid onset of and emergence from the sedated state. In the hands of an experienced anesthesiologist or anesthetist, the depth of anesthesia can be tailored throughout the procedure. Lighter sedation allows for spontaneous breathing and evaluation of airway dynamics. Deeper sedation can be used when performing a BAL and/or other interventional procedures in the lower airways (biopsies).[10–12]

The ideal venue for bronchoscopic procedures is an endoscopy suite or an operating room with continuous cardiopulmonary monitoring, that is fully equipped to manage any foreseeable emergencies, including pulmonary hemorrhage or cardiac arrest.[9] Alternatively, emergency bronchoscopic procedures can be performed at the bedside in the intensive care units (ICUs) with appropriate support from the ICU staff.[13]

WHAT DO YOU NEED TO KNOW BEFORE PERFORMING A FLEXIBLE BRONCHOSCOPY?

RISK FACTORS FOR COMPLICATIONS

An important aspect of preparation is to identify risk factors for complications and to take all necessary actions to prevent them from happening. There are no absolute contraindications to bronchoscopy, although the risks from both the procedure and anesthesia need to be carefully and independently considered for each patient. Flexible bronchoscopy is an invasive procedure and is commonly indicated in patients with chronic and/or complicated comorbidities. There is a risk of complications arising during and after the procedure, so the bronchoscopist should analyze which patients are at higher risk of complications and should determine the appropriate period of observation following the procedure (Tables 2.2, 2.3, and 2.4).[3,4,7,8,14–16]

PERFORMING FLEXIBLE BRONCHOSCOPY: STEPS AND TECHNIQUE

Preparation of the Patient[8–10]

- The patient must be adequately prepared for the procedure; standards differ depending on whether the procedure is performed in the ICU or the OR, and if the procedure is routine or an emergency.
- The patient should be given nothing by mouth (NPO) for a minimum of eight hours for solid food, and four hours for clear liquids in order to decrease the risk of aspiration. These time periods may vary from hospital to hospital. However, emergency procedures may not allow appropriate NPO time, in which case increased precautions should be taken (e.g., rapid anesthesia induction with endotracheal intubation, quick aspiration of stomach contents).
- The patient is placed in a supine position on the procedure table and gently restrained until adequate sedation or anesthesia is achieved.
- The patient should be monitored continuously during the entire procedure, including continuous pulse oximetry and cardiopulmonary monitoring.

Table 2.2 What are the risk factors for flexible bronchoscopy complications?

Risk factor	Conditions	Considerations
Bleeding risk	• Coagulation disorders • Platelet disorder • Sepsis/DIC • Bone marrow transplant • Anticoagulated	• Consult hematology team and provide blood products as needed • Target: Platelet >25,000 or Hb >7.0 • Gentle suction • Be prepared for possible bleeding: cold saline, epinephrine, phenylephrine
Endocrinopathies	• Diabetes mellitus • Adrenal insufficiency • Panhypopituitarism	• Consult endocrinology – clarify need for stress dosing, insulin regimen, and risk of hypoglycemia/hyperglycemia during procedure, same as electrolyte imbalance
Cardiological pathologies	• Pulmonary hypertension • Congenital heart disease • Arrhythmia +/− pacemaker goal	• Consult cardiac anesthesia • Higher risk for hypoxemia, be aware of HR and SpO_2 goals
Aspiration risk	• GI dysmotility risks • TEF, laryngeal cleft suspected • Colonic interposition • Known history of aspiration or abnormal VSS	• May require NPO timing longer than usual • Rapid anesthesia induction
Risk of hypoxia/ Hypoventilation	• Chronic lung disease • Neuromuscular disease • Tracheostomy-Ventilator dependent • Acute respiratory failure	• Provide PPV and oxygen as needed, know baseline ventilator settings and baseline oxygenation need. • Contingency plan should be available

Abbreviations: DIC – Disseminated intravascular coagulation; Hb – Hemoglobin; TEF – Tracheoesophageal fistula; VSS – Video swallow study; GI – Gastrointestinal; HR – Heart rate; NPO – Nothing by mouth; PPV – Positive pressure ventilation

Table 2.3 When to consider hospitalization of a patient for observation after flexible bronchoscopy

Consider observation overnight for:	
Risk factors known before procedure	• Ventilator dependent • Seizure disorder, not well controlled • Immunocompromised/immunosuppressed • Morbid obesity • Complicated endocrinology history – stress dosing, glucose control • Corrected age < 3 months
Findings/ Complications during procedure	• Active pulmonary bleeding visualization • Significant subglottic stenosis, unrepaired • Foreign body removal • Significant purulent bronchitis • Significant hypoxemia/hemodynamical instability • Significant upper airway obstruction, without corrective measurements established (surgical correction, positive pressure ventilation [PPV], tracheostomy)
Post-procedure	• Persistent hypoxemia • Persistent hemodynamic instability • Pneumothorax

Table 2.4 Possible complications of flexible bronchoscopy

Category	Subcategory	Causes	Management
Physiological	Hypoxemia	• Previously known lung disease and airway disease • Sedation (decreased respiratory drive) • Bronchoscope in the airway, causing obstruction • Excessive suctioning/excessive lavage volume	• Provide supplemental oxygen as needed (suction channels, face mask) • Oral airway, laryngeal mask, nasal tube, intubation if needed • Withdraw scope and provide positive pressure
	Hypercapnia/ hypoventilation	• Same causes as hypoxemia	• Withdraw scope and provide positive pressure, allow to improve ventilation • Provide ventilation as needed
	Arrhythmia	• Vagal stimulation due to inadequate anesthesia/ sedation • Hypoxia sensitizes myocardium	• Abort procedure if necessary, allow anesthesia team to intervene • Provide oxygen
	Laryngospasm/ Bronchospasm	• Previously known airway reactivity • Mechanical stimulation of larynx • Inadequate topical anesthesia	• Load with bronchodilators previously or in-procedure through distal filter with closed airway • Systemic steroids in severe cases • Provide adequate anesthesia.
Bacteriological	Iatrogenic infection	• Not following standardized protocol of equipment cleaning	• Treat as needed with antibiotics
	Spread of infection to other areas in the lung	• Lavage of pathologic areas before evaluation of the rest of the lung • Immunocompromised	• Pre-procedural or post-procedural antibiotics to be considered
	Spread of infection to bronchoscopy team	• Airborne agents	• Use PPE as indicated
Mechanical	Pneumothorax	• Procedures – transbronchial biopsy • Inadvertent PEEP (bronchoscope close to inner diameter of artificial airway)	• Thoracostomy set should be available
	Hemorrhage	• Transbronchial biopsy/cytology brush • Advanced bronchiectasis • Airway tumors, pulmonary hypertension, bleeding diastasis	• Possible interventions: epinephrine solution, oxymetazoline, phenylephrine, cold saline, Fogarty catheter, intubated selectively opposite bronchus

(Continued)

Table 2.4 (Continued) Possible complications of flexible bronchoscopy

Category	Subcategory	Causes	Management
	Laryngeal trauma/ Nasal trauma, epistaxis	• Suction trauma, aggressive/fast removal of bronchoscope	• Oxymetazoline pre-bronchoscopy, lubricant, withdraw scope not faster than 5–6 sec, tip NOT held in flexion
	Mucosal edema	• Vigorous suctioning, coughing • Airway collapse around instrument • Intrinsic bronchitis exacerbated	
Anesthesia-related	**Insufficient or excessive anesthesia**	• Vagal stimulation causing laryngospasm/laryngospasm • Decreased respiratory drive – hypoxemia, hypercapnia	• Increase sedation or reverse it as needed by anesthesia team
	Aspiration	• Not adequate NPO timing • Known aspiration risk factors, prevention measurements not taken into account before procedure	• Prevention measures – faster induction, longer NPO, treatment as indicated
Others	**Cardiac arrest**	• Very unlikely – several comorbidities that increase risks of any procedure	• Cardio-respiratory resuscitation

Abbreviations: NP – Nasopharyngeal; ETT – Endotracheal; LMA – Laryngeal mask; PPE – Personal protective equipment; PEEP – Positive end-expiratory pressure; NPO – Nothing by mouth.

- The bronchoscopist typically stands at the head of the table or bed, although bronchoscopy may be performed from the side of the patient, or in any position as necessary.
- If the procedure includes evaluation of the upper airway, oxymetazoline is administered in both nares after the patient has been sedated, then the nose and pharynx are gently suctioned.

"DRIVING" (MANIPULATION) OF THE FLEXIBLE BRONCHOSCOPE: TIPS[17]

- Hand–eye coordination is a priority when driving the flexible bronchoscope to keep the airway centered in the field.
- The handle is grasped with the last three fingers, placing the tip of the thumb on the lever and the first finger over the suction trigger. The shaft of the bronchoscope is held between the thumb and first two fingers of the opposite hand (**Figure 2.8**).
- The tip of the bronchoscope can be flexed or extended in one plane by moving the 'thumb' lever on the control handle. Movement in other planes must be achieved by rotating the shaft of the instrument.
- A loop in the shaft facilitates its rotation and allows better control and precision of the broncho-scope by decreasing the force required to rotate the tip, allowing for > 360 degrees rotation of the tip (**Figure 2.9**).
- The visual field will become totally blocked or blurred when the tip of the scope is against the wall of the airway or has secretions on the lens.
- Sometimes, "the only absolutely reliable anatomic landmark in the upper airways may be the vocal cords" (Robert Wood, MD). When unable to recognize the anatomy, the bronchoscope should be retracted until one can identify reliable landmarks.

- Effective topical anesthesia of the larynx is essential to perform a successful and safe flexible bronchoscopy since direct contact with the laryngeal structures without local anesthesia can result in laryngospasm. Administration of topical anesthesia to the laryngeal structures may cause post-operative aspiration of oral secretions, although the use of a dose of a low-toxicity agent (e.g., lidocaine) minimizes the risk of aspiration.
- A complete airway evaluation starts at the nose; however, the evaluation may start by advancing the scope through a tracheostomy tube, an endotracheal tube, or a laryngeal mask airway (LMA) depending on the specific indications of the procedure and the patient's capacity to maintain appropriate ventilation under anesthesia.

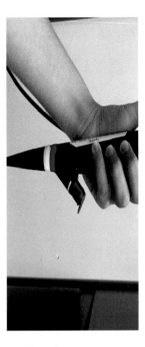

Figure 2.8 Positioning your finger on control handle.

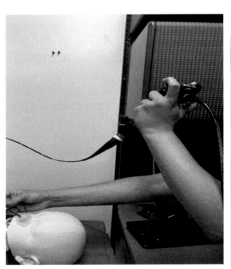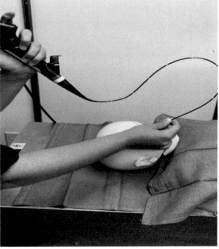

Figure 2.9 Loop to improve rotation of your scope.

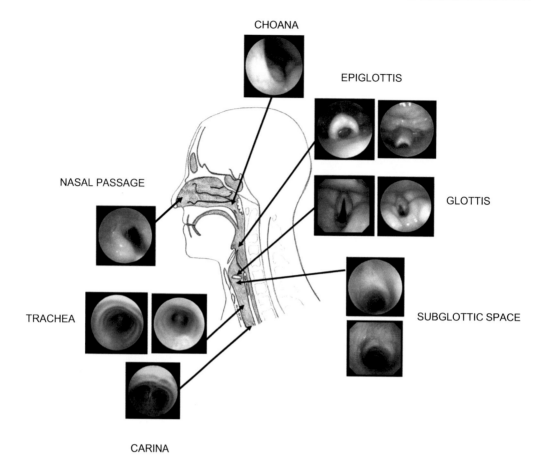

CHOANA

EPIGLOTTIS

NASAL PASSAGE

GLOTTIS

TRACHEA

SUBGLOTTIC SPACE

CARINA

Figure 2.10 Normal upper airway.

- One should be aware that the advancement of a scope through an established airway may result in inadvertent elevation of the positive end-expiratory pressure (PEEP), which could result in the development of a pneumothorax.
- Visualization of the laryngeal structures (Figure 2.10) in patients with an upper airway obstruction can be challenging. To facilitate the evaluation of the structural anatomy, a mandibular lift, or oxygen insufflation, using a flow rate of approximately 2 liters per minute through the suction channel, can be beneficial. However, using these techniques can affect the dynamics of the upper airway.
- Evaluation of the bronchial tree (Figure 2.11) in a systematic way, including all lobar and segmental bronchi, is recommended before obtaining a BAL. The sequence of evaluation is elective.

OBTAINING A BRONCHOALVEOLAR LAVAGE (BAL)[3,18–20]

- Supplies for BAL collection: Sterile specimen trap or sterile syringe, sterile suction tubing, bronchoscope with a suction channel (Figure 2.1).
- BAL sampling technique: Attach the specimen trap to the suction channel, wedge the tip of the bronchoscope in the selected bronchus, ensuring that the suction channel faces the center of the bronchus. Next, inject sterile normal saline through the suction channel, and collect the sample by suctioning gently to avoid traumatizing the mucosa or causing collapse of the bronchial walls. Using a shallow repetitive suction maneuver is usually more effective at obtaining a better fluid return than one long

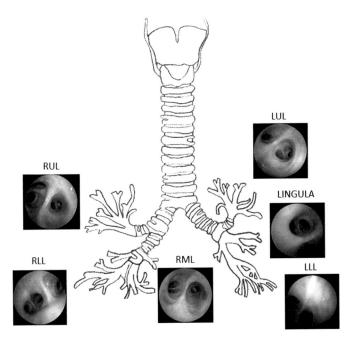

Figure 2.11 Normal lower airway anatomy. RUL: Right upper lobe; RML: Right middle lobe; RLL: Right lower lobe; LUL: Left upper lobe; LLL: Left lower lobe.

sustained suction maneuver. Alternatively, one can use a syringe to manually withdraw the instilled fluid instead of using a mucus trap and suction. The syringe technique results in less suction pressure, therefore creating less collapsing force. This technique is especially useful in patients with severe bronchomalacia or hyperdynamic airway collapse, which can inhibit fluid return.

- The volume of BAL fluid (i.e., sterile normal saline) used should be of sufficient quantity to ensure that some of the effluent sample contains fluid originating from the alveolar space. The instilled volume recommended per BAL aliquot is 5–10 mL in children (approximately 1 mL/kg) and 10–20 mL in adolescents. (Tables 2.5 and 2.6). In these tables, we provide a quick reference for a scope size for specific airway sizes and patient ages.
- The suction port of the flexible bronchoscope is located at 2 o'clock, so is off-center from the video image. Placing the suction channel toward the center of the bronchus lumen and "wedging" the scope when doing BAL are maneuvers that help optimize fluid return.
- After obtaining a BAL sample, orders for processing should be reviewed (Table 2.7).

Table 2.5 Estimated airway size and bronchoscope size[9,14]

Airway size	Scope size
ETT: <3.0 mm	2.2 mm (no O_2 or suction capability, only visualization)
ETT: 3.5–4.0 mm	2.8–3.1 mm (1.2 mm suction channel)
ETT: 4.5 mm	3.7 mm (1.7 mm suction channel)
ETT: 5.0–7.5 mm	4.2–4.4 mm (2.0 mm suction channel)
ETT: >8.0 mm	6.2 mm (2.8 mm suction channel)

Abbreviation: ETT – Endotracheal tube.

Table 2.6 Estimated bronchoscope size based on patient's age

Age	Scope size
< 8 years of age	2.8–3.1 mm (1.2 mm suction channel)
8–14 years of age	3.7 mm (1.7 mm suction channel)
> 14 years of age	4.2–4.4 mm (2.0 mm suction channel)
Adults or adult-sized airways	6.2 mm (2.8 mm suction channel)

Table 2.7 Considerations for diagnostic BAL fluid analysis[3,21]

Patient factors	Orders
Basic BAL orders	• Cytology • Gram stain • Bacterial respiratory culture
Immunocompromised*	• Acid-fast bacterial respiratory culture • Fungal respiratory culture • Galactomannan • Pneumocystis jiroveci • Legionella culture and PCR • Histoplasma antigen and culture • Mycoplasma/Chlamydia PCR • HSV, EBV, CMV, Adenovirus PCR Consider endemic bacteria/fungi in your area+

* Added to Basic BAL orders based on differential diagnosis.
+ By case base scenario
Abbreviations: AFB – Acid fast bacilli; PJP – *Pneumocystis jirovecii*; Ag – Antigen; CF – cystic fibrosis; HSV – Herpes Simplex Virus; EBV – Epstein Barr Virus; CMV Right upper lobe, posterior segment – Cytomegalovirus; PCR – polymerase chain reaction.

POST-BRONCHOSCOPY CARE OF THE PATIENT[17,22–24]

Every sedated patient needs to be monitored and observed until they are awake and back to their baseline status. Patients who have persistent problems post-procedure with hypoxemia, altered mental status, increased work of breathing or difficulties with airway clearance should be observed for a longer period in the post-anesthesia care unit (PACU) or be admitted for observation and monitoring overnight. The level of care necessary at the time of admission will be determined by the patient's clinical status, operative complications, and identified risk factors. (Refer to Tables 2.2, 2.3, and 2.4.)

PROCEDURE REPORT[3]

A detailed procedure report should include:

- Patient identifiers
- Pertinent clinical history
- Indications for the procedure
- Description of the procedure performed
- Complications and amount of blood loss
- Whether BAL was collected, with documentation of labs ordered for BAL
- Description of normal and abnormal findings.
- Discussion, assessment, and plan
- Pictures of important findings can be included in the report

The interpretation of BAL analysis and indicated management recommendations should be added to the procedure report when BAL results become available, including a discussion on how the results support or change the plan previously recommended.

The procedure report should be made available to the referring physician(s) in a timely manner. Images obtained during the evaluation should be reviewed with patients and families and kept with the medical record and/or an electronic bronchoscopy database for future reference.

BRONCHOALVEOLAR LAVAGE SPECIMEN PROCESSING[19]

- *Time for processing* – The BAL sample should be delivered to the lab within one hour of collection
- *Transport to lab* – The BAL sample can be transported *via* a tube system if reliable, but we recommend personally delivering it to the lab (**Figure 2.12**).
- *Minimum quantity of specimen* – At a minimum, 2 mL of the BAL specimen should be collected to ensure adequate sampling, but this should be coordinated according to the minimal sampling required for analysis at your hospital.

NOSOCOMIAL INFECTIONS AND FLEXIBLE BRONCHOSCOPY

Flexible bronchoscopy is a non-sterile aerosol-generating procedure that could become a vector for spreading infectious agents. Infection control measures should be undertaken to prevent nosocomial infections being transmitted to and from the patient, the personnel, the environment, and the equipment. The bronchoscopist and all assistants should each wear a gown, gloves, mask, and goggles. In addition, all used equipment should be handled as potentially infected, being labeled appropriately (clean-dirty) and transported to the cleaning room immediately post-procedure.[3,7,25]

TRANSPORTATION OF THE FLEXIBLE BRONCHOSCOPE

The scope should be transported, preferably in a hard container.

At our hospital, a scope container is used for bronchoscope transport to/from the location of the procedure (procedural room, operating room, or ICU room). A green cover is used to mark as "Clean" (when transporting to the room where the bronchoscopy will occur) and a red cover is used to mark as "Dirty" (when transporting to the cleaning room after use) (**Figure 2.13**).[25]

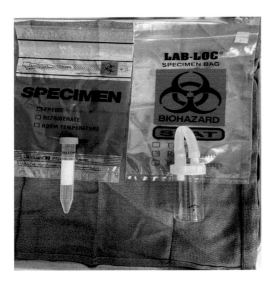
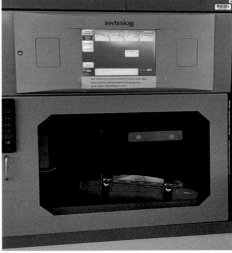

Figure 2.12 Bronchoalveolar lavage transportation.

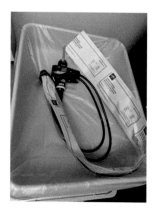
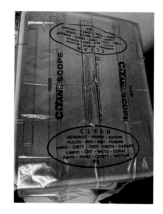
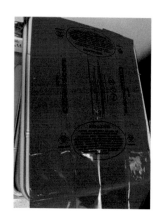

Figure 2.13 Scope containers.

A travel bin is used to transport scopes when the portable cart is used for videorecording of the procedure, e.g., in the ICUs or specialized operating rooms. A label on the outside indicates if the contained scope is "Clean" or "Dirty" (**Figure 2.14**).

CARE OF THE FLEXIBLE BRONCHOSCOPE

Cleaning the Bronchoscope: Infection Control Considerations[25]
The flexible bronchoscope should be cleaned immediately after completing the procedure.

1. Water or saline should be passed under suction through the suction channel to remove gross amounts of blood and secretions, then detergent solution should be passed through the channel under suction.
2. Secretions/blood are wiped from the outside of the bronchoscope with wet gauze or a sponge containing detergent solution.
3. All disposable suction valves and adapters should be removed and discarded.
4. The bronchoscope is transported to the cleaning station in a suitable container.

LEAK TEST[25]

Once the bronchoscope is taken to the sterile processing department (SPD) and before proceeding with the cleaning process, a leak test should be performed by pumping air under pressure through the ethylene oxide valve of the bronchoscope while the instrument is submerged under water.

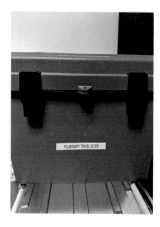
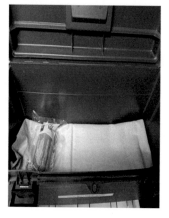
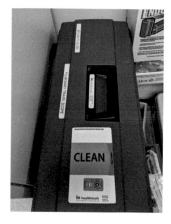

Figure 2.14 Travel bin.

CLEANING AND STERILIZATION[3,7,25,26]

If a leak is identified, the scope is cleaned with enzymatic detergent and processed in the ethylene oxide gas sterilizer before sending it for repair and should not be cleaned with disinfectant solution or through the automatic disinfector.

Instruments free of leaks should be scrubbed inside and out with a brush and soaked in an enzymatic detergent, then rinsed and disinfected. Rinsing can be done by wiping the outside of the scope and suctioning a 70% alcohol solution through the channel. Disinfection can be done manually by submerging the scope in a sterilizing solution (e.g., alkaline glutaraldehyde or 0.55% *ortho*-phthalaldehyde) or by using an automated processing machine. **NEVER put a flexible bronchoscope into an autoclave.**

STORAGE OF THE BRONCHOSCOPE

- Storage of the clean instruments can be achieved by inserting the shaft into a paper sleeve and placing it on a shelf, a drawer or by hanging them from a bracket (**Figure 2.15**). Suction adapters should NOT be attached to the bronchoscope during storage due to the risk of bacterial growth in any residual moisture.

TEAM APPROACH AND BUILDING A BRONCHOSCOPY SERVICE[17,23]

A team is required for appropriate performance of a bronchoscopic examination and is essential for the success and safety of the procedure. The team consists of a physician bronchoscopist, an assistant (i.e., a respiratory therapist or a nurse), an anesthesiologist or a nurse anesthetist, and additional staff to perform the tasks of scheduling, billing, coordination, cleaning and maintenance of the equipment, and housekeeping. The composition of the team may be different in each institution, but the roles listed above must be performed by someone with the skills, training, and support to do the job properly. It is also important to maintain a good

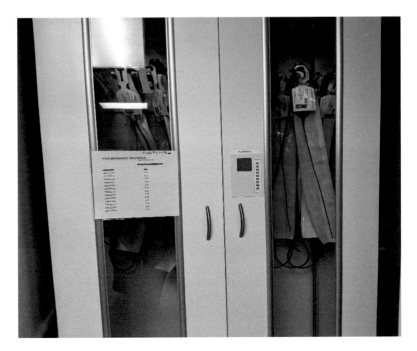

Figure 2.15 Storage of flexible bronchoscopes.

collaborative professional relationship with surgical colleagues, especially professionals skilled in doing rigid bronchoscopy.

The bronchoscopist is the team leader and must be knowledgeable and competent to perform all aspects of the procedure. For bronchoscopy to have a high diagnostic yield and "get the right answer", the bronchoscopist must have knowledge of the differential diagnosis, guide the anesthesiologist on the appropriate level of sedation in a way that allows for an anatomic and dynamic evaluation, appropriately identify normal *versus* abnormal findings, and interpret the findings within the context of the patient's clinical history. All the following aspects should be considered prior to the procedure: (1) indications and risk factors for intraoperative or post-operative complications, (2) urgency of the procedure and patient's clinical stability, (3) availability of the staff, other consulting services, and an appropriate venue for the procedure and post-operative care, and (4) patient/family preferences and expectations.

The endoscopy assistant can be a registered nurse (RN) or a respiratory therapist (RT), depending on the size and philosophy of the institution. The RN or RT typically goes through intense training to collaborate with the physician and nursing staff about the needs for pediatric bronchoscopy and what is clinically indicated for each procedure. Through the team collaboration, the endoscopy assistant is responsible for the equipment, handling of specimens, operation of therapeutic bronchoscopy tools, and assisting in the clinical well-being of the patient.

The anesthesiologist/nurse anesthetist works with the bronchoscopist to deliver an adequate level of sedation that allows for a safe and comfortable diagnostic evaluation while the patient remains breathing spontaneously. Proper communication between anesthesia staff and the bronchoscopist is imperative for the safe management of the airway under conditions that resemble light sleep, which allows for an appropriate evaluation of the airway dynamics and anatomy, leading to the correct diagnosis.

CONCLUSION

In the words of Robert Wood, MD, who is considered to be the father of pediatric flexible bronchoscopy, "The most serious complication, other than death of the patient, is to do the procedure and get the wrong answer". Learning about flexible bronchoscopy is not an easy task but not impossible. Understanding the complications, risk factors, equipment, techniques, and team members needed will give you the information needed to be able to perform the procedure, but practicing it will improve your proficiency, skills, and confidence.

REFERENCES

1. Wood RE. Spelunking in the pediatric airways: explorations with the flexible fiberoptic bronchoscope. *Pediatr Clin North Am.* 1984;31:785–99.
2. Wood RE, Sherman JM. Pediatric flexible bronchoscopy. *Ann Otol Rhinol Laryngol.* 1980;89:414–6.
3. Faro A, et al. Official American Thoracic Society technical standards: flexible airway endoscopy in children; American Thoracic Society Ad Hoc Committee on Flexible Airway Endoscopy in Children. *Am J Respir Crit Care Med.* 2015;191:1066–80.
4. Wood RE, Postman D. Endoscopy of the airways in infants and children. *J Pediatr.* 1988;112:1–6.
5. Gans SL, Berci G. Advances in endoscopy of infants and children. *J Pediatr Surg.* 1971;6:199–233.
6. Gonzalez C, Reilly J, Bluestone CD. Synchronous airway lesions in infancy. *Ann Otol Rhinol Laryngol.* 1987;96:77–80.
7. Green CG, et al. Flexible endoscopy of the pediatric airway. *Am Rev Respir Dis.* 1992;145:223–5.
8. Mahmoud N, Vashisht R, Sanghavi D, et al. Bronchoscopy. [Updated 2021 Jul 31]. In: *StatPearls* [Internet]. Treasure Island, FL: StatPearls Publishing; 2021 Jan. (basics).
9. Wood RE. Bronchoscopy and bronchoalveolar lavage in pediatric patients. In: *Kendig's Disorders of the Respiratory Tract in Children*, 2006;9, 134–46.e1. Elsevier, New York

10. Wood RE, Finke RJ. Application of flexible fiberoptic bronchoscopes in infants and children, *Chest*. 1978;73(Supplement):737–40.

11. Cote CJ. Sedation for the pediatric patient. A review. *Pediatr Clin North Am*. 1994;41:31–58.

12. Cote CJ, Wilson S, American Academy of Pediatrics, American Academy of Pediatric Dentistry. Guidelines for monitoring and management of pediatric patients before, during, and after sedation for diagnostic and therapeutic procedures. *Pediatrics* June 2019; 143 (6): e20191000.

13. Efrati O, et al. Flexible bronchoscopy and bronchoalveolar lavage in pediatric patients with lung disease. *Pediatric Crit Care Med*. 2009;10:80–4.

14. Linnane B, Hafe GM, Ranganathan SC. Diameter of pediatric sized flexible bronchoscopes: when size matters. *Pediatric Pulmonol*. 2006;41:787–9.

15. Credle WF, et al. Complications of fiberoptic bronchoscopy. *Am Rev Resp Dis*. 1974;109:67–72.

16. Albertini Re, HJH, et al. Arterial hypoxemia induced by fiber-optic bronchoscopy. *JAMA*. 1974;230:1666–7.

17. Wood, R. Chapters 6 and 7. Techniques of flexible bronchoscopy in infants and children. In: *Pediatric Flexible Bronchoscopy*. A postgraduate Course. Cincinnati, OH, 09/10-13/2019, 2019;6:1–6:15.

18. Baughman RP. Technical aspects of bronchoalveolar lavage: recommendations for a standard procedure. *Semin Resp Crit Care Med*. 2007;28:475–85.

19. de Blic J, Midulla F, Barbato A, et al. Bronchoalveolar lavage in children. ERS Task Force on bronchoalveolar lavage in children. European Respiratory Society. *Eur Respir J*. 2000;15:217–31.

20. Reynolds HY. Bronchoalveolar lavage. *Am Rev Respir Dis*. 1987;135:250–63.

21. Pattishall EN, Noyes BE, Orenstein DM. Use of bronchoalveolar lavage in immunocompromised children with pneumonia. *Pediatr Pulmonol*. 1988;5:1–5.

22. Wood RE. Pitfalls in pediatric flexible bronchoscopy. *Chest*. 1990;97:199–203.

23. Welshe S, et al. Pediatric bronchoscopy. Special considerations. *AORN J*. 1987;46:864–8.

24. Committee on Drugs. American Academy of Pediatrics. Guidelines for monitoring and management of pediatric patients during and after sedation for diagnostic and therapeutic procedures. *Pediatric*. 1992;89:110–5, and addendum Pediatrics. 110: 836-8, 2002.

25. Mehta AC, Prakash UBS, Garland R, et al. American College of Chest Physicians and American Association for Bronchoscopy consensus statement: prevention of flexible bronchoscopy-associated infection. *Chest*. 2005;128:1742–55.

26. Rutala WA, Weber DJ. FDA labeling requirements for disinfection of endoscopes: a counterpoint. *Infect Control Hosp Epidemiol*. 1995;16:231–5.

3

Basics of microlaryngoscopy and rigid bronchoscopy

CAROL LI, GREGORY BURG, AND KARA D. MEISTER

INTRODUCTION

Microdirect laryngoscopy and rigid bronchoscopy are useful in a wide array of clinical scenarios and are often utilized in conjunction with flexible bronchoscopy and esophagogastroduodenoscopy in the evaluation of aerodigestive complaints. In particular, microdirect laryngoscopy and rigid bronchoscopy are optimal for the diagnosis of posterior laryngeal clefts and tracheoesophageal fistulas. Furthermore, these techniques can be therapeutic, such as in foreign body removal from an airway or for management of large-volume bleeding. Rigid bronchoscopy should be considered as being complementary to flexible bronchoscopy, as should the collaboration between pulmonology, otolaryngology, and the anesthesia or intensivist teams. This chapter will summarize the key principles and practical guidelines for setting up and performing microdirect laryngoscopy and rigid bronchoscopy in the operating room setting. The order of these procedures is important, as a shallow depth of anesthesia is critical to an accurate display of dynamic function during flexible bronchoscopy and rigid bronchoscopy, when possible. Therefore, multidisciplinary aerodigestive evaluations are performed in order from the least anesthesia to the deepest anesthesia in a structured fashion, ideally with a dedicated team of anesthesia colleagues sensitive to these nuances. More details regarding multidisciplinary aerodigestive evaluation are described in Chapter 9.

DOI: 10.1201/9781003106234-3

RIGID BRONCHOSCOPES

Rigid bronchoscopes were first developed in the early twentieth century. The rigid bronchoscope is superior for the evaluation of the anatomy of the upper and central airways. Its rigid nature allows for probing and movement of structures, which helps to facilitate the identification of clefts, fistulas, scar tissue formation, etc. These instruments have excellent optics and allow for positive pressure ventilation of the patient during the procedure. The rigid bronchoscopes are sized according to their internal diameter, which is relatively large and facilitates the passage of a wide variety of instruments while maintaining ventilation and direct visualization of the airway.

ADVANTAGES OF RIGID BRONCHOSCOPY

- Capacity to remove foreign bodies
- Capacity to perform surgical interventions through the scope (e.g., cautery)
- Better visualization of the posterior wall of the glottis, subglottis, and cervical trachea
- Capacity to probe airway structures, allowing for greater diagnostic yield of laryngo-esophageal cleft, tracheoesophageal fistula (TEF), and fixation by scarring of the supraglottic and/or glottic structures

PREPARATION

A successful and efficient airway evaluation in the operating room is dependent upon preparation, equipment availability, personnel, and room arrangement. Pediatric rigid bronchoscopy is most often carried out in the operating room and occasionally in other clinical locations, such as the intensive care unit or cardiac catheterization laboratory, when necessary.

ANESTHESIA

An open and constant line of communication should occur between the anesthesia and surgical teams as the responsibility for airway management is frequently shared. The patient should be maintained in a plane of anesthesia deep enough to tolerate the procedure, ideally with spontaneous ventilation.

- Consider administration of systemic steroids, such as a one-time dose of dexamethasone 0.5 mg/kg up to 8–10 mg for airway edema. Antibiotics are not generally indicated for diagnostic procedures.
- Supplemental oxygenation can be provided by nasal cannula, high-flow nasal cannula/THRIVE™, or insufflation into the upper airway *via* an endotracheal tube (ETT) positioned in the hypopharynx. Some laryngoscopes also have ports for the insufflation of oxygen. Additionally, if a rigid ventilating bronchoscope is used, this will adapt for use with the anesthesia circuit for assisted ventilation.

ROOM ARRANGEMENT

After induction of general anesthesia, the patient should be turned 90 degrees from the anesthesiologist with the head toward the surgeon (**Figure 3.1**). The instrument table and video input tower should be positioned adjacent to the surgeon. Monitors with the endoscopic view, as well as the patient's vital signs, should be in view.

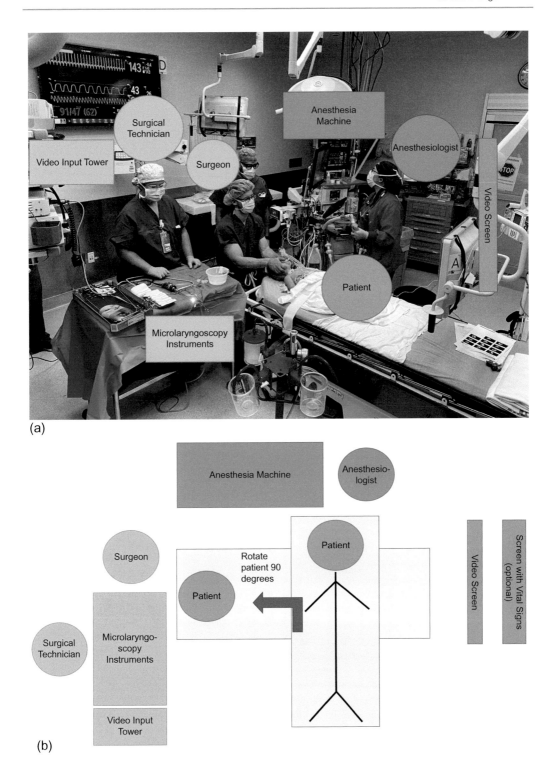

Figure 3.1 Operating room layout: real view (a) and schematic (b).

PATIENT FACTORS

Optimal patient positioning is critical for effective direct laryngoscopy and rigid bronchoscopy. The patient should be supine and positioned up at the head of the operating table. The head and neck should start in a neutral position. A pillow or towel roll can be used to stabilize the patient's head and prevent it from rolling to the side. The chest should be exposed to detect respiratory effort and adequate ventilation. Gastrostomy tubes should be ventilated, unless specifically evaluating for trachea-esophageal fistulas.

EQUIPMENT

Prior to the procedure beginning, surgical safety time-out and equipment checks should be performed.

- It is often advisable to have two suctions available and turned on.
- Video monitors for the endoscopy feed and the vital signs should be visible to both the bronchoscopy team and the anesthesia team.
- Necessary equipment includes tools to expose, examine, palpate, measure, and photo/video document the examination. Our basic setup comprises a variety of laryngoscopes, bronchoscopes, zero degree and angled telescopes, a right-angle probe, a vocal fold spreader, rigid and flexible suctions, and uncuffed ETTs. For a complete airway examination, the following instruments and medications should be on the procedure table (Figure 3.2):
  - Dental guard
  - Laryngoscope
  - Topical anesthesia (e.g., lidocaine) with atomizer
  - Rigid endoscope (bronchoscopy)
  - Light source
  - Camera head
  - Endotracheal tubes
  - Normal saline/sterile normal saline
  - Anti-fog solution
  - Gauze/microwipe
  - Suction (rigid and flexible)
  - Alligator forceps

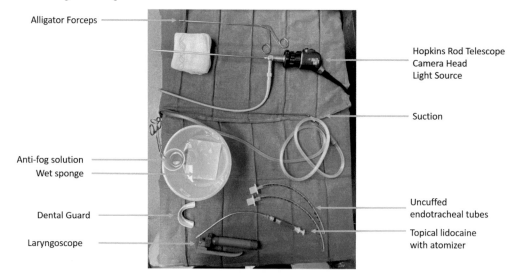

Figure 3.2 Microlaryngoscopy and bronchoscopy instruments.

TECHNIQUE

After the patient is turned 90 degrees from the anesthesia team, the surgeon takes over control of the airway and begins to mask the patient, with the use of a jaw thrust to keep the airway open, if necessary. Confirming the ability to mask the patient with a tolerance of jaw thrust and persistence of patient-initiated breaths indicates a proper depth of anesthesia. The upper dentition or alveolus should be inspected and then protected with a dental guard or gauze, respectively. The dental guard may be trimmed with scissors to accommodate the child's oral cavity.

- The mouth is opened in a scissors technique to expose the oral cavity and tongue.
- The oral cavity, oropharynx, hypopharynx, larynx, and esophageal inlet are examined with microdirect laryngoscopy.
  - The laryngoscope, such as a Philips or a Wisconsin blade, is positioned according to the shape of the laryngoscope. In children, a straight blade laryngoscope placed in the vallecula most often affords a view of the laryngeal inlet while allowing atraumatic passage of the bronchoscope.
  - Factors such as individual preference and experience, equipment availability, and airway anatomy may be considered when choosing the appropriate blade; there are no definitive data which consider one style to be superior to the other.[1]
- An age-appropriate laryngoscope is passed into the oral cavity with the blade to the right of the tongue and used in a sweeping motion to direct the tongue leftward while passing the tip of the blade into the vallecula. Having a second light handle available in case of dimming is advisable, as well as a backup style of blade.
- The laryngoscope is pulled upward and anteriorly to impart traction to the glossoepiglottic ligament and lift the epiglottis, thus exposing the glottic inlet.
- Once the airway is in view, passive insufflation of oxygen should be provided – it is the author's preference to use a 3.5 or 4.0 uncuffed ETT placed in the left hypopharynx and incorporated into the surgeon's left hand, which also holds the laryngoscope and the patient's jaw.
- Topical anesthetic (lidocaine) is then atomized onto the vocal folds to prevent laryngospasm (if this was not already performed during the preceding flexible bronchoscopy). The dose depends upon the child's weight.
- The use of a rigid telescope can provide a shared, magnified view and affords video and photo documentation. A rigid Hopkins rod telescope is then introduced, and standard photo documentation of the supraglottis, glottis, subglottis, trachea, and bilateral mainstem bronchi is carried out (Video 3.1, Figure 3.3).

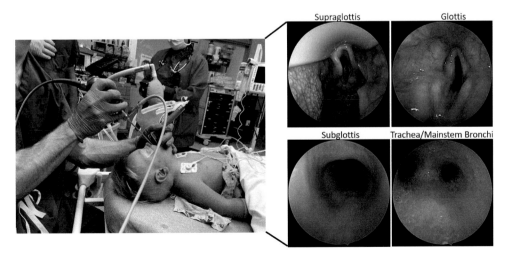

Figure 3.3 Microlaryngoscopy and bronchoscopy technique with standard photo documentation of the supraglottis, glottis, subglottis, trachea, and bilateral mainstem bronchi.

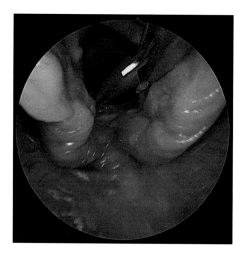

Figure 3.4 Palpation of a laryngoesophageal cleft using alligator forceps.

- It is our practice to begin with a 0° 4 mm × 18 cm Hopkins rod-lens telescope for routine evaluations.
- In very small infants, children with suspected airway stenosis, or those at risk of needing urgent intubation, which may benefit from visualizing placement into the airway, a smaller telescope may be needed (0° 2.7 mm × 18 cm or 0° 1.9 mm × 11.5 cm). A 2.5 or 3.0 ETT placed over the smaller telescope can be used in a Seldinger technique to facilitate urgent intubation (it may be necessary to remove the ETT connector in advance to facilitate placement of the ETT over the telescope without overhang at the distal end).
- If the larynx needs to be examined or operated upon with a two-hand technique, the patient can be placed into laryngeal suspension.
- The difficulty and grade of exposure is noted, and the laryngoscope used is documented in the electronic medical record and in the operative report for quick reference. External laryngeal manipulation by the surgeon or an assistant can often improve a difficult view.
- The supraglottis and glottis are examined and photo documented. A right-angle probe (or alligator forceps) is used to evaluate for laryngeal cleft and to palpate for a submucous cleft of the posterior cricoid, and a photo is captured in all patients to document this portion of the examination (**Figure 3.4**). The cricoarytenoid joints are also palpated with the instrument to check for mobility.
- The subglottis is sized with progressive intubation of uncuffed ETTs and examined for a leak by endoscopic visualization of air (**Video 3.2**).
- The trachea is then visually inspected for tracheoesophageal fistula, complete tracheal rings, inflammation, and tracheobronchomalacia/compression. Both rigid and flexible bronchoscopy can provide data regarding the degree of tracheal collapse and malacia, given that dynamic, spontaneous ventilation is maintained.[2,3]
- Attention is turned to the segmental and subsegmental bronchi. Turning the head to the opposite side of the bronchi (e.g., to examine the bronchus intermedius, turn the patient's head to the left) facilitates passage of the scope and other instruments into the distal airway.
- It is our practice to examine the same basic battery of structures in every patient, with additional examination based on the patient's history and pre-operative diagnostic workup.

Video 3.1 This is an example of a rigid bronchoscopy performed on a child using a Hopkins rod and spontaneous ventilation. The alligator forceps are used to examine the interarytenoid space for a possible laryngeal cleft.

Video 3.2 With an endotracheal tube in the airway, just beyond the subglottis, positive pressure is uptitrated while examining for a visible leak of air around the endotracheal tube.

USE OF THE RIGID VENTILATING BRONCHOSCOPE

Using only the Hopkins rod to perform the airway evaluation has the significant advantage of decreased airway resistance relative to the larger-sized ventilating bronchoscope. The disadvantage, however, is that the telescope alone does not provide any ability to ventilate or secure the airway. In cases of suspected foreign body or children with poor pulmonary reserve, the use of the ventilating bronchoscope should be considered rather than the Hopkins rod.

Technique

- Exposure of the larynx is performed *via* direct laryngoscopy, as described above.
- The bevel should be turned 90 degrees counterclockwise while passing into the subglottis in order not to injure the true vocal folds.
- Once the bronchoscope is endotracheal, the laryngoscope can be removed, and the corresponding hand can transition to the patient's forehead with a finger on the patient's palate to provide a base for the bronchoscope. The bronchoscope is then stabilized with the left hand, with one finger on the patient's hard palate acting as the scope's base and fulcrum
- The anesthesia circuit can then be connected. The accordion adaptor will ameliorate tension from the circuit, but, if it is lost or falls, the anesthesia circuit can connect to the ventilation port on the bronchoscope.
- The diagnostic evaluation can then proceed as previously described. If the patient becomes hypoxic or hypercarbic, the telescope and suction can be removed to provide a larger-caliber airway; the broncho-scope should be blocked off by the glass cap or a gloved finger. Additionally, a larger-caliber suction can be passed through the rigid bronchoscope if the telescope is removed.
- The reader is referred to Chapter 9 for further discussion of therapeutic interventions with rigid bron-choscopy, such as foreign body removal or management of hemoptysis.

Special patient populations and techniques

- 22q11.2-deletion syndrome: Special attention is paid to palpation of the palate and examination for glot-tic web, as well as tracheobronchomalacia secondary to vascular compression.[4] Examination of a glottic web should include visualization of the subglottic component with an angled telescope.
- Children with a history of VACTERL, CHARGE, or other midline defects should be carefully evaluated for TEF.
- Esophageal atresia/tracheoesophageal fistula (EA-TEF): It is our practice to perform rigid bronchos-copy on every patient with newly diagnosed EA-TEF in coordination with pediatric surgery.[5,6] Children with a history of tracheoesophageal fistula and with wheezing or stridor should be evaluated for other midline anomalies of the aerodigestive tract, such as laryngeal cleft and recurrent fistula.[7] A high index of suspicion of synchronous airway anomalies, such as complete tracheal rings or significant tracheo-malacia, should be maintained in all patients with EA-TEF.[8]

Complications and D-disposition

- Complications of rigid bronchoscopy are dependent upon multiple factors, including patient anatomy and comorbidities, indications for the procedure, clinical setting, equipment factors, anesthesia-related factors, and provider and institutional experience.
- The most common complications are related to the placement of rigid instrumentation and include gum/dental injury, lip pinching/lacerations, pharyngeal lacerations, laryngeal edema, and laryngospasm/bronchospasm.[9]

- Pneumothorax and barotrauma can occur if there is over-insufflation or with the use of high suction pressures with high airway pressures. A vasovagal response can also be elicited with the use of the bronchoscope; this may be more pronounced in infants < six months of age.[10]
- Rarely, direct injury to the trachea or bronchus from the telescope or bronchoscope can result in pneumothorax or subcutaneous emphysema.
- Cognitive failures also occur when the bronchoscopist misses or does not appreciate pathology.
- Following rigid bronchoscopy for diagnostic purposes, most patients can be discharged on the same day, following an observation period in the post-anesthesia care unit (disposition following therapeutic interventions can differ widely, however).

Pearls

- If exposure cannot be achieved with the laryngoscope, a rigid bronchoscope can be used to enter the airway. The ventilating bronchoscope is passed down the right glossotonsillar sulcus, posteriorly along the posterior pharyngeal wall, and lifts the epiglottis directly for a view of the glottis.
- Evaluation of tracheoesophageal fistula, either primary, recurrent, or iatrogenic, can be done by gently placing a cuffed ETT into the esophagus and gently insufflating the esophagus with air while visualizing the trachea endoscopically. Gently pulling the ETT proximally can evaluate the posterior tracheal wall. Close communication with anesthesia is imperative to prevent over-insufflation of the esophagus. The stomach should be decompressed following this examination.

CONCLUSION

Bronchoscopy is crucial to the evaluation of the upper airway in pediatric patients. Investigation of upper airway pathology relies upon both flexible and rigid endoscopy and requires clinicians trained in the techniques and interpretations of findings of both modalities. Ideally, these clinicians are collaborating in a multidisciplinary, concurrent approach. Performing a comprehensive evaluation of the upper airway requires clinical expertise, procedural skill, and a safe environment with appropriate equipment and support staff. Flexible bronchoscopy, rigid bronchoscopy, and hybrid techniques are often complementary with distinct and overlapping indications for the evaluation of the upper airway.

TIPS FOR CLINICAL PRACTICE

- In a smaller patient with retrognathia or an otherwise anterior larynx, gripping the laryngoscope between the thumb and palm of the hand can leave the pinky finger free to provide anterior laryngeal/cricoid pressure for better exposure, when an assistant is not available.
- Use a light touch with the laryngoscope so as to not distort the anatomy unnecessarily. Cupping the child's head with the left hand can facilitate the examination. Holding the laryngoscope off to a slight angle can also open the aperture to allow easier passage of the telescope and instruments.
- The smallest ventilating rigid bronchoscope which will accommodate instrumentation is the 3.5; it is advisable to start with a ventilating bronchoscope of at least size 3.5, if feasible.
- A hybrid technique of passing a flexible bronchoscope through a rigid ventilating bronchoscope can facilitate specific scenarios, such as foreign bodies in the distal airway or pathology of hard-to-access areas, such as the right upper lobe bronchus.[11]

REFERENCES

1. Matuszczak M, Gooden CK. Direct laryngoscopy equipment and techniques. In: Jagannathan N, Fiadjoe JE, editors. *Management of the Difficult Pediatric Airway* [Internet]. 1st ed. Cambridge University Press; 2021 [cited 2020 Dec 30]. p. 27–37. Available from: https://www.cambridge.org/core/product/identifier/9781316658680%23CN-bp-4/type/book_part

2. Choi J, Dharmarajan H, Yu J, Dunsky KA, Vece TJ, Chiou EH, et al. Diagnostic flexible versus rigid bronchoscopy for the assessment of tracheomalacia in children. *J Laryngol Otol.* 2018 Dec;132(12):1083–7.

3. Hysinger EB, Hart CK, Burg G, De Alarcon A, Benscoter D. Differences in flexible and rigid bronchoscopy for assessment of tracheomalacia. *Laryngoscope.* 2021 Jan;131(1):201-204.

4. Wong NS, Feng Z, Rappazzo C, Turk C, Randall C, Ongkasuwan J. Patterns of dysphagia and airway protection in infants with 22q11.2-deletion syndrome. *Laryngoscope.* 2020 Nov;130(11):2532–2536.

5. Baxter KJ, Baxter LM, Landry AM, Wulkan ML, Bhatia AM. Structural airway abnormalities contribute to dysphagia in children with esophageal atresia and tracheoesophageal fistula. *J Pediatr Surg.* 2018 Sep;53(9):1655–9.

6. Parolini F, Morandi A, Macchini F, Canazza L, Torricelli M, Zanini A, et al. Esophageal atresia with proximal tracheoesophageal fistula: A missed diagnosis. *J Pediatr Surg.* 2013 Jun 1;48(6):e13–7.

7. Thakkar HS, Hewitt R, Cross K, Hannon E, De Bie F, Blackburn S, et al. The multi-disciplinary management of complex congenital and acquired tracheo-oesophageal fistulae. *Pediatr Surg Int.* 2019 Jan 1;35(1):97–105.

8. Wolter NE, Kennedy AA, Rutter MJ, Matava C, Honjo O, Chiu PL, et al. Diagnosis and management of complete tracheal rings with concurrent tracheoesophageal fistula. *Int J Pediatr Otorhinolaryngol.* 2020 Jun 1;133:109971.

9. Chaddha U, Murgu S. Complications of rigid bronchoscopy. *Respirology.* 2021 Jan;26(1):14–8.

10. Van Beek-King JM, Rastatter JC. Rigid bronchoscopy equipment and techniques. In: Jagannathan N, Fiadjoe JE, editors. *Management of the Difficult Pediatric Airway* [Internet]. 1st ed. Cambridge University Press; 2021 [cited 2020 Dec 30]. p. 112–7. Available from: https://www.cambridge.org/core/product/identifier/9781316658680%23CN-bp-10/type/book_part

11. Singhal KK, Singh M, Kanojia RP, Mathew JL, Vaidya PC, Pandey A. Flexible through rigid bronchoscopy for airway foreign body: A good marriage of convenience! *Pediatr Pulmonol [Internet].* [cited 2020 Dec 30];n/a(n/a). Available from: http://onlinelibrary.wiley.com/doi/abs/10.1002/ppul.25167

4

Upper airway bronchoscopic interpretation

ANITA DESHPANDE, CHERIE A. TORRES-SILVA, AND CATHERINE K. HART

INTRODUCTION

This chapter describes the anatomy of the upper airway, from the nasal cavity to the carina, and is structured according to the anatomic order in which these structures are encountered when performing flexible or rigid bronchoscopy. A systematic approach to assessing each anatomic subsite facilitates the identification of abnormalities in an efficient and effective manner. Flexible and rigid endoscopy of the upper airway are complementary and are ideally performed together to provide a comprehensive evaluation of the upper airway. Clinical symptoms, interpreted within the clinical context of each individual patient, should guide the bronchoscopist's differential diagnosis and elevate the index of suspicion for certain anatomic abnormalities. The reader is also referred to Chapter 2, **Figure 2.11**.

NASAL CAVITY

Upper airway evaluation usually starts by inserting an endoscope, either a flexible bronchoscope or a nasal endoscope, into the nasal cavity. In the clinical context of nasal obstruction and/or obstructive sleep apnea, the bronchoscopist should focus particular attention on anatomic sources of obstruction, including the septum, the internal nasal valve, and the external nasal valve. Topical medications, which often contain a mixture of local anesthetic and decongestant, can affect and underestimate the contribution of mucosal edema to nasal obstruction. Endoscopic examination should start at the internal nasal valve, which is formed by the septum, the head of the inferior turbinate, and the caudal border of the upper lateral cartilage. This is

DOI: 10.1201/9781003106234-4

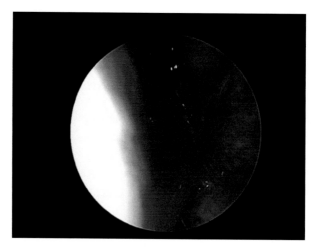

Figure 4.1 Choanal atresia.

typically the narrowest portion of the nasal cavity, and endoscopic assessment should make note of both static structural abnormalities, such as septal deviation, spur, or inferior turbinate hypertrophy, as well as dynamic collapse, due to weakness of the upper lateral cartilage that can occur during inspiration.[1] Once past the internal nasal valve, the middle turbinate comes into view. Lateral to the middle turbinate is the middle meatus, into which the anterior ethmoid, maxillary, and frontal sinuses drain. Common pathology at this site can include polyps or mucopurulent drainage. Moving posteriorly, the choana, or opening between the nasal cavity and nasopharynx, is encountered. Choanal atresia, or lack of formation of this opening, can be unilateral or bilateral. This deformity can be comprised of bony, membranous, or mixed atresia, and clinical presentation can vary, from acute airway obstruction if bilateral choanal atresia is present to unilateral chronic nasal obstruction and rhinorrhea.[2] Evaluation of this condition should occur by passing the endoscope through both nasal cavities to assess for patency (**Figure 4.1**).

NASOPHARYNX

The nasopharynx extends from the skull base to the inferior extent of the soft palate. In the nasopharynx, a common cause of obstruction in children is adenoid hypertrophy (**Figure 4.2**). Adenoid tissue usually

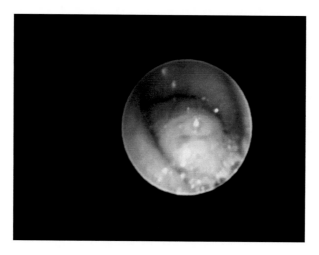

Figure 4.2 Adenoid hypertrophy.

involutes during adolescence,[3] but persistence into adulthood can represent a variety of pathological conditions, such as allergy or an immunodeficiency syndrome.[4] A variety of benign and malignant tumors can also occur at this site, though they are rare in the pediatric population. Benign lesions include fibroma, chordoma, nasal dermoid, encephalocele, nasal glioma, teratoma, craniopharyngiomas, and Thornwaldt's cyst.[5] Malignant lesions include rhabdomyosarcoma, nasopharyngeal carcinoma, and lymphoma.[5] Abnormal tissue in this area should prompt referral to an otolaryngologist for evaluation and management, likely to include cross-sectional imaging.

SOFT PALATE

Next, the soft palate, or velum, is encountered. The velum, lateral pharyngeal walls, and posterior pharyngeal wall form the velopharyngeal valve, which separates the nasopharynx from the oropharynx. Closure of this valve is essential during functions such as speech and swallowing[6] and is accomplished through the contraction of several muscles (e.g., the levator veli palatini, musculus uvulae, etc.). Notation should be made of soft palate closure patterns, which are important in the evaluation of obstructive sleep apnea and velopharyngeal insufficiency. These patterns are characterized by coronal closure, sagittal closure, circular closure, and circular closure with Passavant's ridge.[7,8] The orientation of the palate should be noted, as well as the presence of clefting or a bifid uvula.

ORAL CAVITY AND OROPHARYNX

When evaluating the posterior oral cavity and oropharynx, the endoscopist should take care to identify the palatine tonsils and their size and contribution to oropharyngeal collapse (**Figure 4.3**). Glossoptosis and lingual tonsillar hypertrophy (**Figure 4.4**) are also important in the evaluation of obstructive sleep apnea. With the flexible endoscope in place just inferior to the soft palate, a jaw thrust maneuver should be performed to assist in differentiation between these two conditions, as jaw thrust should improve an obstruction caused by glossoptosis (**Figure 4.5**). Symmetry of the vallecula should also be assessed. Masses located at the base of the tongue can include a lingual thyroglossal duct cyst (**Figure 4.6**) or a lingual thyroid, either of which can cause potential airway displacement and subsequent respiratory distress.[9]

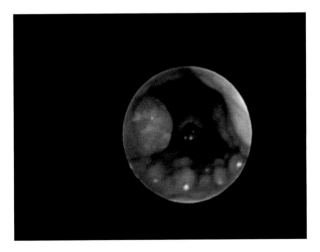

Figure 4.3 Palatine tonsil hypertrophy.

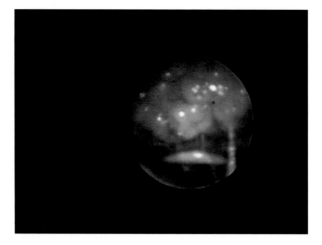

Figure 4.4 Lingual tonsillar hypertrophy.

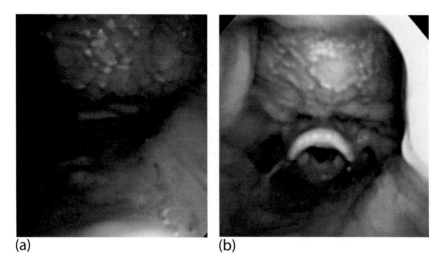

(a) (b)

Figure 4.5 Glossoptosis: (a) without jaw thrust; (b) with jaw thrust.

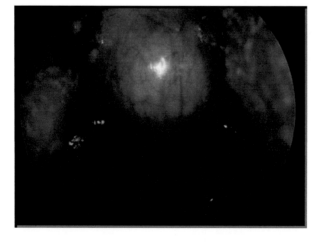

Figure 4.6 Lingual thyroglossal duct cyst.

HYPOPHARYNX

The postcricoid region comprises the anterior wall of the hypopharynx. There is a rich venous plexus in this area, which can become engorged during the expiratory phase of an infant's cry. Engorgement of this area, which can occur with bluish-purple vascular discoloration, is termed the postcricoid cushion and is hypothesized to protect against emesis.[10] Postcricoid masses, such as mucus retention cysts,[11] lymphovascular malformations,[12] sarcoidosis,[13] and amyloidosis,[14,15] occur primarily in adults and are rare in the pediatric population.[16]

EPIGLOTTIS AND SUPRAGLOTTIC LARYNX

Airway malacia, which includes laryngomalacia, tracheomalacia, and bronchomalacia, is a dynamic obstruction of the airways and is the most common congenital airway anomaly in children. Laryngomalacia is a condition in which supraglottic structures, including the aryepiglottic folds, the arytenoid, corniculate, or cuneiform cartilages, the epiglottis, or a combination of all the above, collapse into the larynx and obstruct airflow during inspiration (Video 4.1). Flexible bronchoscopy *via* a trans-nasal approach during spontaneous ventilation allows for thorough dynamic evaluation. Common findings include shortened aryepiglottic folds, an omega-shaped epiglottis, and redundant arytenoid mucosa that can prolapse into the larynx.[17]

Video 4.1 Laryngomalacia.

LARYNX

The endoscope is then brought closer in order to examine the vocal cords in greater detail. Vocal nodules are the most common cause of dysphonia in children[18] and typically appear as firm, bilateral lesions located medially along the membranous vocal fold.[19] Polyps are generally unilateral and can be sessile or pedunculated. Cysts can be categorized as mucoid or epidermoid and can be found along the medial edge of the membranous vocal fold or infracordal. Granulomas are often associated with mucosal trauma, such as intubation, surgical defect, or chronic cough, and are usually located in the vocal process.[20] Recurrent respiratory papillomatosis is a challenging disease to control, can cause significant morbidity, and, in rare cases, can undergo malignant transformation.[21] These lesions appear as recurrent, exophytic papillomas within the respiratory tract (Figure 4.7).

It is also important to evaluate the patient for a deep interarytenoid notch or a laryngotracheoesophageal cleft, especially in children with a history of aspiration. This is best performed with the rigid bronchoscope held in position above the glottis with an assistant palpating the interarytenoid area with a suction probe or alligator forceps in order to assess the interarytenoid depth relative to vocal cord position.[22]

SUBGLOTTIS

The subglottis is the narrowest portion of the neonatal airway and is bounded by the cricoid ring. Congenital subglottic stenosis results from a failure of recanalization of the larynx during embryogenesis and can present as small glottic webs, lateral elliptical shelving, or complete laryngeal atresia.[23,24] The cricoid is a complete ring of cartilage that can be prone to circumferential injury with resultant scarring, such as from prolonged intubation of premature infants during the neonatal period, which can thus result in acquired subglottic

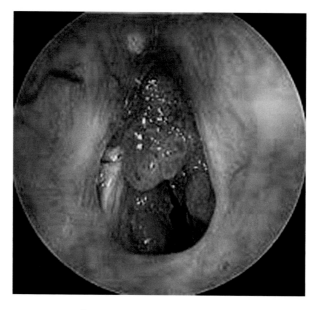

Figure 4.7 Recurrent respiratory papillomatosis.

stenosis (**Figure 4.8**).[25] When subglottic stenosis is encountered, airway size should be determined. The size of the subglottic area is determined by identifying the size of an endotracheal tube that will pass through the stenotic area and tolerate normal leak pressures (10–25 cm H_2O). The measured size should be compared with the expected age-appropriate endotracheal tube size in order to grade the degree of stenosis.[26]

The subglottis can also be involved with several neoplastic lesions. Hemangiomas are the most common tumors of the infant subglottis.[27] They are generally not present at birth, but they present and proliferate rapidly within weeks to months of birth. The proliferative phase usually lasts for 6 to 12 months and is then followed by an involution phase that can be variable in length. On endoscopy, these lesions present as a smooth,

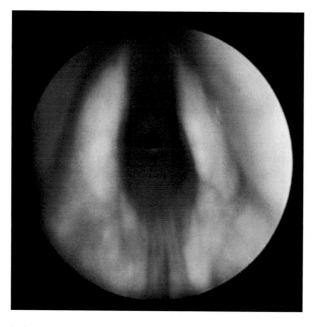

Figure 4.8 Grade III subglottic stenosis.

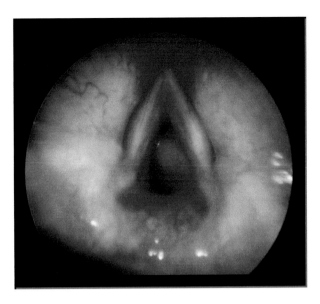

Figure 4.9 Subglottic cyst.

submucosal swelling, more commonly located on the left side of the subglottis and posteriorly. They may also demonstrate blanching with pressure.

Subglottic cysts, which can be congenital or acquired, are retention cysts of the subepithelial mucosal glands and also commonly arise in the posterolateral subglottis (Figure 4.9).[28] They can be associated with prematurity and intubation in the early neonatal period.[29] They can be treated endoscopically with decompression, excision, or marsupialization[30] or by using laser, microdebrider, or coblator.[29] Following treatment, surveillance endoscopic examinations should be performed to assess for recurrent cyst formation.[28]

Malignant tumors of the pediatric airway are very rare. These can include squamous cell carcinoma, rhabdomyosarcoma, and mucoepidermoid carcinoma, among others.

PROXIMAL TRACHEA

The endoscope is then advanced further to evaluate the trachea. Tracheomalacia is the most common congenital anomaly of the trachea and is diagnosed with endoscopy performed with the patient spontaneously breathing (Video 4.2). Flexible bronchoscopy may allow for a more thorough evaluation of malacia as rigid bronchoscopes may artificially stent open the trachea. Greater than 50% narrowing of the airway lumen is considered to be diagnostic of tracheomalacia.[31] Vascular compression should also be noted, as tracheal compression can result from vascular anomalies or congenital heart defects.[31]

Video 4.2 Tracheomalacia.

Complete tracheal rings are the most common cause of tracheal stenosis.[32] This anomaly is characterized by the absence of a membranous trachea and the trachealis muscle. The cartilaginous rings of the affected trachea are circular and smaller than an unaffected trachea (Figure 4.10).

The bronchoscope should be withdrawn, with careful attention being paid to the posterior tracheal wall to evaluate for a tracheoesophageal fistula (TEF). Tracheoesophageal fistulas can be congenital, in which there is abnormal development of the tracheoesophageal septum, or can be acquired, as with trauma or malignancy.[33,34] In children with a history of aspiration or recurrent pneumonia, great care should be taken to assess

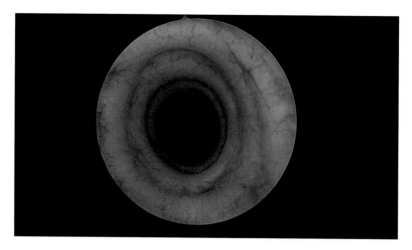

Figure 4.10 Complete tracheal rings.

for a TEF. On bronchoscopy, a TEF can occasionally appear as a very obvious connection between the trachea or esophagus, but, more commonly, a TEF appears as a subtle dimple or discoloration in the mucosa or as a more prominent groove.[35] In some instances, the pouch that remains after TEF ligation can contain a persistent TEF which can be difficult to visualize. The use of a flexible bronchoscope to probe a TEF pouch (e.g., using air insufflation to blow open a small fistula) or an area of dimpling along the posterior tracheal wall can help to identify subtle TEFs that would be difficult to visualize with rigid bronchoscopy alone (**Video 4.3**).

Video 4.3 Probing of the tracheoesophageal fistula (TEF) pouch.

CONCLUSION

The upper airway is best evaluated systematically by each anatomic subsite with both rigid and flexible endoscopy. This comprehensive approach facilitates the identification of abnormalities. Clinical context guides the interpretation of bronchoscopic findings.

TIPS FOR CLINICAL PRACTICE

- Assess each anatomic subsite for abnormalities
- Some abnormalities are best identified using rigid bronchoscopy, such as laryngeal clefts
- Some abnormalities are best identified using flexible bronchoscopy, such as airway malacia in some patients

REFERENCES

1. Patel B, Virk JS, Randhawa PS, Andrews PJ. The internal nasal valve: a validated grading system and operative guide. *Eur Arch Otorhinolaryngol.* 2018 Nov;275(11):2739–44. doi: 10.1007/s00405-018-5142-x. Epub 2018 Oct 6. PMID: 30293091; PMCID: PMC6208712.
2. Kwong KM. Current updates on choanal atresia. *Front Pediatr.* 2015 Jun 9;3:52. doi: 10.3389/fped.2015.00052. PMID: 26106591; PMCID: PMC4460812.

3. Handelman CS, Osborne G. Growth of the nasopharynx and adenoid development from one to eighteen years. *Angle Orthod.* 1976 Jul;46(3):243–59. doi: 10.1043/0003-3219(1976)046<0243:GOTNAA>2.0.CO;2. PMID: 1066976.

4. Merati AL, Rieder AA. Normal endoscopic anatomy of the pharynx and larynx. *Am J Med.* 2003 Aug 18;115(Suppl 3A):10S–14S. doi: 10.1016/s0002-9343(03)00187-6. PMID: 12928069.

5. Birkeland AC, McHugh JB, Bohm LA. A pediatric nasopharyngeal mass. *JAMA Otolaryngol Head Neck Surg.* 2018 Apr 1;144(4):371–2. doi: 10.1001/jamaoto.2017.3072. PMID: 29392294.

6. Perry JL. Anatomy and physiology of the velopharyngeal mechanism. *Semin Speech Lang.* 2011 May;32(2):83–92. doi: 10.1055/s-0031-1277712. Epub 2011 Sep 26. PMID: 21948636.

7. Croft CB, Shprintzen RJ, Rakoff SJ. Patterns of velopharyngeal valving in normal and cleft palate subjects: a multi-view videofluoroscopic and nasendoscopic study. *Laryngoscope.* 1981 Feb;91(2):265–71. doi: 10.1288/00005537-198102000-00015. PMID: 7464388.

8. Finkelstein Y, Shapiro-Feinberg M, Talmi YP, Nachmani A, DeRowe A, Ophir D. Axial configuration of the velopharyngeal valve and its valving mechanism. *Cleft Palate Craniofac J.* 1995 Jul;32(4):299–305. doi: 10.1597/1545-1569_1995_032_0299_acotvv_2.3.co_2. PMID: 7548102.

9. Zimmerman KO, Hupp SR, Bourguet-Vincent A, Bressler EA, Raynor EM, Turner DA, Rehder KJ. Acute upper-airway obstruction by a lingual thyroglossal duct cyst and implications for advanced airway management. *Respir Care.* 2014 Jul;59(7):e98–e102. doi: 10.4187/respcare.02513. Epub 2013 Oct 29. PMID: 24170914; PMCID: PMC4331108.

10. Hoff SR, Koltai PJ. The "postcricoid cushion": observations on the vascular anatomy of the posterior cricoid region. *Arch Otolaryngol Head Neck Surg.* 2012 Jun;138(6):562–71. doi: 10.1001/archoto.2012.932. PMID: 22710508.

11. Sidell D, Joshi AS, Kieliszak CR, Bielamowicz SA. Isolated lymphatic malformation of the postcricoid space. *Ear Nose Throat J.* 2018 Aug;97(8):E52–E53. doi: 10.1177/014556131809700813. PMID: 30138530.

12. Smith NM, Stafford FW. Post cricoid lymphangioma. *J Laryngol Otol.* 1991 Mar;105(3):220–1. doi: 10.1017/s0022215100115427. PMID: 2019814.

13. Vaz FM, Samuel D. Postcricoid sarcoid mimicking a malignancy: a lesson to remember. *Otolaryngol Head Neck Surg.* 2000 Jul;123(1 Pt 1):150. doi: 10.1067/mhn.2000.107394. PMID: 10889500.

14. Chadwick MA, Buckland JR, Mason P, Randall CJ, Theaker J. A rare case of dysphagia: hypopharyngeal amyloidosis masquerading as a post-cricoid tumour. *J Laryngol Otol.* 2002 Jan;116(1):54–6. doi: 10.1258/0022215021910140. PMID: 11860656.

15. Bhavani RS, Lakhtakia S, Sekaran A, Tandan M, Reddy ND. Amyloidosis presenting as postcricoid esophageal stricture. *Gastrointest Endosc.* 2010 Jan;71(1):180–1; discussion 181. doi: 10.1016/j.gie.2009.08.013. PMID: 19836745.

16. Contrera KJ, Elsheikh TM, Hopkins B, Hadford S, Anne S. Benign postcricoid hypertrophy: case report and review of the literature. *Int J Pediatr Otorhinolaryngol.* 2020 Nov;138:110308. doi: 10.1016/j.ijporl.2020.110308. Epub 2020 Aug 13. PMID: 32846331.

17. Hysinger EB. Laryngomalacia, tracheomalacia and bronchomalacia. *Curr Probl Pediatr Adolesc Health Care.* 2018 Apr;48(4):113–8. doi: 10.1016/j.cppeds.2018.03.002. Epub 2018 Apr 3. PMID: 29622320.

18. Mudd P, Noelke C. Vocal fold nodules in children. *Curr Opin Otolaryngol Head Neck Surg.* 2018 Dec;26(6):426–30. doi: 10.1097/MOO.0000000000000496. PMID: 30300211.

19. Hron TA, Kavanagh KR, Murray N. Diagnosis and treatment of benign pediatric lesions. *Otolaryngol Clin North Am.* 2019 Aug;52(4):657–68. doi: 10.1016/j.otc.2019.03.010. Epub 2019 May 11. PMID: 31088693.

20. Jang M, Basa K, Levi J. Risk factors for laryngeal trauma and granuloma formation in pediatric intubations. *Int J Pediatr Otorhinolaryngol.* 2018 Apr;107:45–52. doi: 10.1016/j.ijporl.2018.01.008. Epub 2018 Jan 31. PMID: 29501310.

21. Derkay CS. Recurrent respiratory papillomatosis. *Laryngoscope.* 2001 Jan;111(1):57–69. doi: 10.1097/00005537-200101000-00011. PMID: 11192901.

22. Ojha S, Ashland JE, Hersh C, Ramakrishna J, Maurer R, Hartnick CJ. Type 1 laryngeal cleft: a multidimensional management algorithm. *JAMA Otolaryngol Head Neck Surg.* 2014 Jan;140(1):34–40. doi: 10.1001/jamaoto.2013.5739. PMID: 24263209.

23. Hanlon K, Boesch RP, Jacobs I. Subglottic stenosis. *Curr Probl Pediatr Adolesc Health Care.* 2018 Apr;48(4):129–35. doi: 10.1016/j.cppeds.2018.03.007. PMID: 29801771.

24. Milczuk HA, Smith JD, Everts EC. Congenital laryngeal webs: surgical management and clinical embryology. *Int J Pediatr Otorhinolaryngol.* 2000 Jan 30;52(1):1–9. doi: 10.1016/s0165-5876(99)00284-0. PMID: 10699233.

25. Jagpal N, Shabbir N. Subglottic stenosis. 2020 Oct 12. In: *StatPearls* [Internet]. Treasure Island, FL: StatPearls Publishing; 2021 Jan. PMID: 33085412.

26. Myer CM 3rd, O'Connor DM, Cotton RT. Proposed grading system for subglottic stenosis based on endotracheal tube sizes. *Ann Otol Rhinol Laryngol.* 1994 Apr;103(4 Pt 1):319–23. doi: 10.1177/000348949410300410. PMID: 8154776.

27. Ida JB, Guarisco JL, Rodriguez KH, Amedee RG. Obstructive lesions of the pediatric subglottis. *Ochsner J.* 2008 Fall;8(3):119–28. PMID: 21603463; PMCID: PMC3096332.

28. Chandran A, Sagar P, Kumar R, Shreshtha N. Addressing a rare cause of paediatric stridor: subglottic cyst. *BMJ Case Rep.* 2020 Jun 28;13(6):e236600. doi: 10.1136/bcr-2020-236600. PMID: 32595124; PMCID: PMC7322319.

29. Agada FO, Bell J, Knight L. Subglottic cysts in children: a 10-year review. *Int J Pediatr Otorhinolaryngol.* 2006 Aug;70(8):1485–8. doi: 10.1016/j.ijporl.2006.03.010. Epub 2006 May 2. PMID: 16650484.

30. Bowles PFD, Reading J, Albert D, Nash R. Subglottic cysts: The Great Ormond Street experience in 105 patients. *Eur Arch Otorhinolaryngol.* 2021 Jun;278(6):2137–41. doi: 10.1007/s00405-020-06321-z. Epub 2020 Sep 1. PMID: 32875392.

31. Carden KA, Boiselle PM, Waltz DA, Ernst A. Tracheomalacia and tracheobronchomalacia in children and adults: an in-depth review. *Chest.* 2005 Mar;127(3):984–1005. doi: 10.1378/chest.127.3.984. PMID: 15764786.

32. Rutter MJ, Cotton RT, Azizkhan RG, Manning PB. Slide tracheoplasty for the management of complete tracheal rings. *J Pediatr Surg.* 2003 Jun;38(6):928–34. doi: 10.1016/s0022-3468(03)00126-x. PMID: 12778396.

33. Ng TY, Kirimli BI, Datta TD. Unrecognized tracheo-oesophageal fistula. *Anaesthesia.* 1977 Jan;32(1):31–3. doi: 10.1111/j.1365-2044.1977.tb11554.x. PMID: 322530.

34. Reed WJ, Doyle SE, Aprahamian C. Tracheoesophageal fistula after blunt chest trauma. *Ann Thorac Surg.* 1995 May;59(5):1251–6. doi: 10.1016/0003-4975(94)00964-9. PMID: 7733742.

35. Wong MD, Gauld LM, Masters IB. Flexible bronchoscopy in diagnosis and management of dual tracheoesophageal fistula: a case series. *Clin Case Rep.* 2020 Jun 16;8(9):1765–8. doi: 10.1002/ccr3.2978. PMID: 32983492; PMCID: PMC7495836.

5

Lower airway bronchoscopic interpretation

KIMBERLEY R. KASPY AND SARA M. ZAK

INTRODUCTION

Evaluation of the lower airways *via* flexible bronchoscopy is an important diagnostic tool in understanding pulmonary pathophysiology.[1] This chapter describes the normal anatomy and typical abnormalities of the airways below the glottis that may be encountered during flexible bronchoscopy. Indications and advantages of assessing the lower airways with a flexible instrument will first be discussed, followed by describing the normal anatomy and interpretation of common pathology of the lower airways.

There are several indications for endoscopic evaluation of the lower airways with a flexible bronchoscope, including but not limited to chronic cough, unexplained or persistent wheezing, recurrent pneumonia, persistent radiographic opacities, microbiological sampling, and suspected airway compression or obstruction, among others.[1] Depending on the indication for the procedure, flexible bronchoscopy can be used to assess airway dynamics in addition to airway anatomy and to collect a sample for culture and cytology with bronchoalveolar lavage.[2] There are many instances where flexible bronchoscopy is performed in conjunction with rigid bronchoscopy, with this portion generally performed by pediatric otolaryngology. Flexible bronchoscopy can be done *via* the natural airway (i.e., through the nose/mouth) or through an artificial airway, such as a laryngeal mask airway (LMA) or an endotracheal tube (ETT). Flexible bronchoscopy in children is generally performed in the operating room with sedation by anesthesia or in the intensive care unit (ICU) with sedation administered by the ICU team.[1]

DOI: 10.1201/9781003106234-5

ADVANTAGES OF FLEXIBLE BRONCHOSCOPY OVER RIGID BRONCHOSCOPY FOR EVALUATION OF THE LOWER AIRWAYS

The indications for flexible and rigid bronchoscopy in pediatric patients often overlap, although there are several advantages to evaluating the lower airways with a flexible bronchoscope rather than a rigid bronchoscope. First, the flexible bronchoscope is able to assess more distal airways than rigid instruments and can better assess the upper lobe segments.[3] Because it can reach more distally, the flexible bronchoscope is the preferred instrument for obtaining bronchoalveolar lavage sampling.[2] Second, the flexible scope can be passed through an artificial airway, including tracheostomy tubes, ETTs, or LMAs, and can be used to assess the lower airways in patients who have limited jaw/mandibular opening.[1,3,4] Third, the flexible instrument can better assess airway dynamics as it allows the patient's airway to remain in a more natural position, as opposed to using a laryngoscope with significant neck extension for rigid bronchoscopy, which puts traction on the larynx and can distort dynamics.[3]

Limitations to flexible bronchoscopy for evaluation of the lower airways may include obstructing the lumen of the airway, particularly if using an artificial airway, and a small suction channel.

PEARLS

- Endoscopic evaluation of the pediatric lower airways should be performed by a provider with appropriate training and experience, as it is not without risk.[1]
- It is important to have a standardized approach to assessing the airways to ensure that all portions are evaluated in order to avoid missing pathology. All pertinent imaging and lab results should be reviewed prior to the procedure.
- The endoscopist should be positioned in a spot where they are comfortable for the duration of the procedure (often at the head of the bed or to the side of the patient's head) and where they can safely maintain the airway of the patient throughout the procedure.
- A trained bronchoscopy assistant should be present to set up the equipment and assisting with obtaining and handling specimens.[1]
- If assessing the lower airways through an artificial airway, it is important to have the correct-sized bronchoscope that will fit through. Of note, the smallest endotracheal tube a 2.8 mm bronchoscope will safely fit through is a 3.5 mm endotracheal tube. Please refer to Chapter 2 for a summary of appropriate bronchoscope/airway sizing.
- If obtaining a bronchoalveolar lavage for infectious etiologies, reasonable attempts at delaying antibiotic administration should be made, as cultures may quickly become sterilized. There are times when this is not possible, and cytology can still be useful to provide information regarding possible causes. Interpretation of bronchoalveolar lavage is discussed further in Chapter 7.
- Photo imagery and video documentation of the clinical findings are strongly encouraged as images can often provide a more comprehensive understanding of findings and can be used for reference and comparison.

NORMAL LOWER AIRWAY ANATOMY

The lower airways consist of the trachea, bronchi, bronchioles, and alveoli. Only the trachea, lobar, and segmental and proximal sub-segmental bronchi are able to be evaluated with a flexible bronchoscope. Please refer to **Figure 5.1a–e** for normal endoscopic imaging of the lower airways.

TRACHEA

- The trachea is a long cylindrical tube, with C-shaped cartilage rings covering approximately 300 degrees of the anterior wall and a posterior trachealis muscle.[5,6]

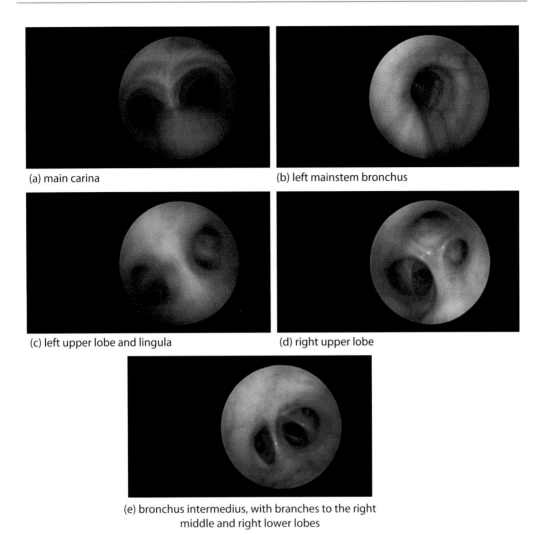

(a) main carina

(b) left mainstem bronchus

(c) left upper lobe and lingula

(d) right upper lobe

(e) bronchus intermedius, with branches to the right middle and right lower lobes

Figure 5.1 (a–e) Normal endoscopic imaging of the lower airways.

- The posterior trachealis is membranous and mobile but, during quiet breathing, should not show significant intrusion into the airway
- The trachea ends at the carina, where it bifurcates into the right and left mainstem bronchi.

BRONCHI

- At the distal end of the trachea, the airways bifurcate into the right and left mainstem bronchi.
- The bronchi have a similar structure to the trachea, with cartilage rings forming the anterior wall and a posterior membranous portion. The cartilage extends into the segmental bronchi and will disappear at the level of the bronchioles (which cannot be visualized *via* endoscopy).
- The right mainstem bronchus has a more straight-line bifurcation from the carina than the left. There are three lobar bronchi in the right lung – the right upper lobar bronchus, the right middle lobar bronchus, and the right lower lobar bronchus.[7]
    - The right upper lobe generally takes off shortly after the carina. There are generally three segmental bronchi in the right upper lobe – the anterior, posterior, and apical.
    - The right middle and lower lobes take off from the bronchus intermedius.
    - The right middle lobe has two segmental bronchi – the medial and lateral bronchi.

 – The right lower lobe has four basilar segments – the medial, anterior, lateral, and posterior. There is also a superior segment of the right lower lobe that generally takes off just distal to the right middle lobe on the opposite side of the bronchus intermedius.

- The left mainstem bronchus divides into two lobar bronchi – the left upper lobe and the left lower lobe. The left lung take-off is at a much more acute angle than the right mainstem bronchus, with a longer distance to the lobar bronchi, which generally cannot be seen from the carina.[7]
    – The left upper lobe divides into the apical-posterior and anterior segments and the lingular segments (superior and inferior).
    – The left lower lobe has a superior segment and three basilar segments, namely the anteromedial, lateral, and posterior segments.

Pearls

- When evaluating the lower airways, keep the tip of the bronchoscope in the center of the airway, off the walls. Try to avoid advancing blindly; suggestions to clear the tip of the bronchoscope include gentle suction, instilling a few milliliters of saline in the suction channel, or wiping the tip of the bronchoscope on a mucosal surface. If you do not know where you are in the lower airways, retract the scope until you reach a point where you can re-establish your location.
- It is important to be able to identify normal lower airway and segmental bronchi anatomy in order to be able to recognize abnormalities.
- There is typically variability in the lower lobe segmental bronchi anatomy bilaterally; the above is considered a guide, but additional imaging (such as CT or fluoroscopy) can help identify the segmental bronchi more definitively.
- The right upper lobe can occasionally take off before the carina; this is referred to as a tracheal (or pig) bronchus. There may also be two right upper lobes – one tracheal bronchus with one to two segments and another distal to the carina in its typical location. Please refer to **Figure 5.2** for the endoscopic appearance of a tracheal bronchus. This is a normal anatomic variant and is generally considered to be an incidental finding.[5]
- Patients with complete situs inversus will have "flipped" or reversed anatomy – the typical structures of the right-sided airways will be seen on the patient's left, with typical left-sided airways on the patient's right. Patients with situs ambiguous can have left isomerism with bilobed lungs bilaterally or right isomerism with trilobed lungs bilaterally. These findings can be associated with primary ciliary dyskinesia or congenital heart disease.[7,8]

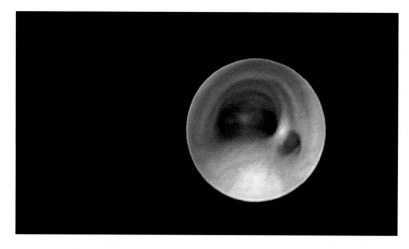

Figure 5.2 Endoscopic appearance of a tracheal bronchus.

COMMON LOWER AIRWAY ABNORMALITIES

Lower airway pathology can be located at any level of the tracheobronchial tree. Abnormalities can be either congenital or acquired at any point in life. Examples of acquired causes include intubation, surgical interventions, or infections; for some findings causes will be briefly explored in this section but not explored in detail. This section will discuss commonly seen structural and dynamic abnormalities, starting in the trachea and then in the bronchi.

SUBGLOTTIS

The subglottis is the uppermost portion of the trachea, just below the vocal cords but above the thoracic inlet. In pediatric patients, the cricoid cartilage is the narrowest portion of the airway compared to the vocal cords of adults.

- The most common lesion seen in the subglottis is subglottic stenosis (SGS).[9] This can be congenital or acquired. The most common cause of acquired subglottic stenosis in pediatric patients is trauma/injury due to prolonged intubation.[8,10]
- Subglottic stenosis is graded based on the degree of narrowing in the airway, called the Cotton-Myer grading system.[11]
    - Grade 1 SGS is less than 50% narrowing of the subglottis
    - Grade 2 SGS is 51%–70% narrowing of the subglottis
    - Grade 3 SGS is 71%–99% narrowing of the subglottis (seen in Figure 5.3a)
    - Grade 4 SGS results when there is no detectable opening into the distal trachea, which is depicted in Figure 5.3b

TRACHEA

- *Tracheoesophageal fistula (TEF)*
    - This is an abnormal connection between the trachea and esophagus and can be congenital or acquired, though it is more commonly congenital. There are several variations of TEF, which may be associated with esophageal atresia (EA).[12] Children with EA and TEF will present at birth, whereas H-type TEF or isolated TEF (without EA) can present later in life.
    - The most common type of TEF is associated with distal EA, in which the upper esophagus ends in a blind pouch, and the distal esophagus arises from the distal trachea. In this case, on endoscopy the lower esophagus may appear like an extra bronchus just above or near the carina (Figure 5.4a). Following repair, there is generally a residual pouch at the site of the prior fistula (shown in Figure 5.4b).[12]

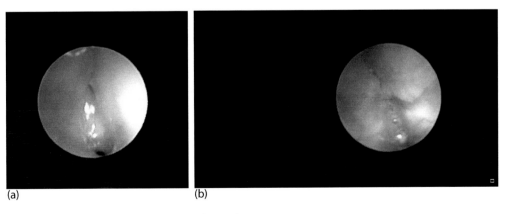

(a)   (b)

Figure 5.3 Subglottic stenosis (a) grade III (b) grade IV.

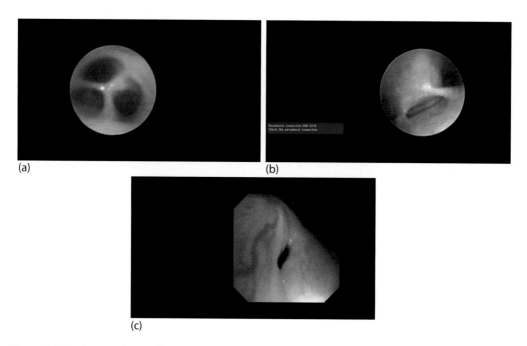

(a)　　　　　　　　　　　　　　　　(b)

(c)

Figure 5.4 Tracheoesophageal fistula (TEF). A TEF is shown at the level of the carina (a). Following repair, there is often a residual pouch at the site of the prior fistula (b). An H-type TEF is a slit-like opening in the posterior tracheal wall that opens into and connects to the esophagus (c).

- An H-type TEF is associated with essentially normal tracheal and esophageal anatomy; in this type, there is a slit-like opening in the posterior tracheal wall that opens into and connects to the esophagus (**Figure 5.4c**).
- *Laryngeal cleft*
  - This is a congenital abnormality where there is an abnormal connection between the trachea and the esophagus (similar to TEFs) from an opening in the posterior laryngotracheal wall. However, in this case, the posterior membrane of the trachea and the anterior wall of the esophagus did not form normally, resulting in a common tube for both the trachea and esophagus.[13,14]
  - Types 1 and 2 clefts occur at the level of the glottis, with Type 1 being the mildest (Type 1 is a gap to the vocal cords but above the cricoid cartilage, with Type 2 extending below the vocal cords into the cricoid cartilage). Types 3 and 4 extend into the trachea, with Type 4 being the most severe form, which can extend down to the mainstem carina (Type 3 extends through the cricoid cartilage into the cervical trachea and Type 4 extends further down the trachea below the thoracic inlet).[13] A Type 4 laryngeal cleft is shown in **Video 5.1**.
  - These can be difficult to diagnose *via* flexible bronchoscopy and are typically better evaluated with a rigid bronchoscope.
- *Tracheal stenosis*
  - Tracheal stenosis involves significant narrowing of the trachea. The most common cause is congenital complete tracheal rings,[15,16] in which the tracheal cartilage forms a complete ring (as opposed to the typical ~300 degree C-shaped ring) as shown in **Figure 5.5**. Congenital tracheal stenosis can present with life-threatening respiratory failure and often requires surgical intervention.[17] Complete tracheal rings can characteristically be associated with cardiovascular anomalies such as pulmonary artery sling or with trisomy 21.
  - Acquired tracheal stenosis can occur from prolonged intubation, infection, or inflammation.[17]
  - Idiopathic tracheal stenosis can occur in pediatric patients but is generally seen in adult women.[17,18] This can involve small sections of the trachea or the entire trachea.

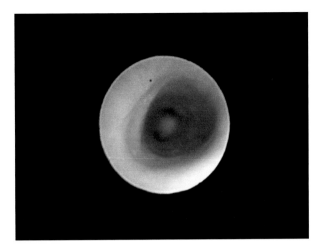

Figure 5.5 Congenital tracheal stenosis caused by complete tracheal rings.

- *Tracheomalacia*
  - This is a condition of excessive dynamic collapse of the trachea during the respiratory cycle. There is no standardized classification system of the degree of tracheomalacia seen, though it is often described when the airway lumen is reduced by > 50%, with severe tracheomalacia generally associated with > 90% reduction in the lumen.[19–21] The presence of tracheomalacia on bronchoscopy can be very dependent on the level of anesthesia and how forcefully the patient is breathing during the procedure.
  - In patients with tracheomalacia, the tracheal rings do not extend for the normal ~300 degrees and are often shorter and/or flattened. This results in a broader, posterior tracheal wall, which will then protrude into the airway with expiration, leading to narrowing of the tracheal lumen, as shown in **Video 5.2**. This will worsen with more forceful exhalation and coughing.
  - Tracheomalacia can be localized to a small section of the trachea or extend for nearly the entire length of the trachea. It is most commonly seen near the end of the trachea before it branches into the mainstem bronchi and is often associated with bronchomalacia.
- *Tracheal compression*
  - Compression of the trachea is described when there is a narrowing of the tracheal lumen caused by external compression of the trachea. This is typically the result of other structures in the mediastinum, such as large blood vessels and vascular rings/slings.[22–24]
  - The anterior wall of the trachea is most commonly affected by external compression, with the innominate artery and the aorta being the most common vessels that cause tracheal compression. An example of tracheal compression is shown in **Video 5.3**.
  - When compression is due to a large blood vessel, the compression may appear pulsatile, though lack of pulsatility does not exclude vascular compression.
- *Tracheal obstruction*
  - The trachea can also be subjected to obstruction, whether from a foreign body or from intraluminal lesions. Foreign body removal is discussed in Chapter 9 and should generally be performed in conjunction with a rigid bronchoscopy by pediatric otolaryngology.
  - **Figure 5.6** demonstrates respiratory papillomatosis, caused by the human papilloma virus (HPV). This virus causes wart-like lesions in the airway, generally beginning in the upper airway/larynx, but can spread down into the lower airway. As there is a risk of malignant transformation of these lesions, it is important that they are closely monitored and treated. Potential endoscopic interventions for treatment are discussed in Chapter 9.
  - Sarcomas and other cancerous lesions can be found in the airway and can cause obstruction, though these are rare in children.[25]
  - Subglottic hemangiomas and cysts can also cause obstruction in the upper trachea.

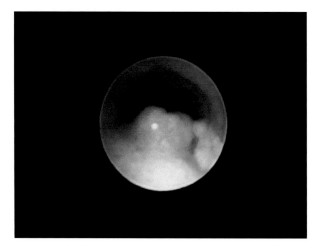

Figure 5.6 Recurrent respiratory papillomatosis.

- *Tracheopathy*
  - The mucopolysaccharidoses (MPS), such as Hunter's syndrome and Hurler's syndrome, can cause tracheopathies, in which substances are deposited within the airway mucosa because they cannot be digested by the body.
  - These deposits can lead to tracheal distortion and stenosis over time. Depending on the severity of the disease, this tracheopathy can extend throughout the airway and into the bronchi, leading to worsening narrowing of the airway.
  - Management of these patients is further discussed in Chapter 9.
- *Tracheal cartilaginous sleeve*
  - This is a rare congenital malformation where the tracheal rings are replaced by a segment of continuous cartilage leading to narrowing of the airway.
  - Most commonly, tracheal cartilaginous sleeves have been described in patients with syndromic craniosynostosis such as Crouzon, Pfeiffer, and Apert syndromes.[26]
- *Tracheostomy tubes*
  - Acquired structural tracheal deformities can occur secondarily to having a tracheostomy tube.
  - A tracheostomy tube, while necessary for breathing in patients that have them, is a foreign object in the airway and can lead to granulation tissue production, both above the stoma as well as at the distal end of the tube.
  - Inflated tracheostomy cuffs can also cause erosion or irritation to the tracheal mucosa.
  - Many patients who undergo tracheostomy placement can acquire tracheal stenosis at their stoma site, due to the collapse of a cartilage ring. This is often referred to as an A-frame tracheal deformity, named according to the shape it forms in the airway. This is shown in **Figure 5.7**.

 Video 5.1 Laryngeal cleft.

 Video 5.2 Tracheomalacia.

 Video 5.3 Tracheal compression.

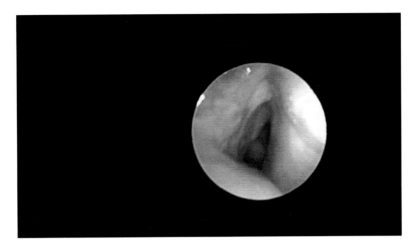

Figure 5.7 A-frame tracheal deformity, named due to the shape it forms in the airway.

PEARLS

- H-type TEFs can be difficult to diagnose with flexible bronchoscopy and may be better seen with rigid bronchoscopy.
- Distinguishing between tracheomalacia and tracheal compression can be difficult. Tracheomalacia tends to be more dynamic, generally occurring during the expiratory phase of breathing, and will worsen with heavier breathing or coughing. Tracheal compression generally occurs anteriorly with compression of the anterior tracheal wall, whereas tracheomalacia occurs from the protrusion of the posterior tracheal membrane into the tracheal lumen.
- Many tracheal anomalies are associated with underlying syndromes (such as VATER, VACTERL, CHARGE, trisomy 21), which may warrant additional evaluation.

BRONCHIAL TREE

- *Bronchial stenosis* is a narrowing of the lumen of the bronchi.
  - Chronic infection and inflammation, such as from a retained foreign body, can lead to scarring and narrowing of a bronchial lumen (seen in **Figure 5.8**).

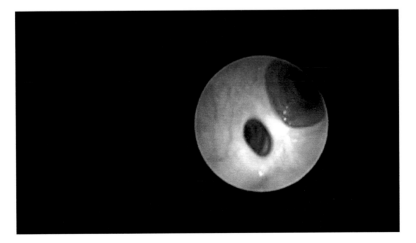

Figure 5.8 Chronic infection and inflammation, such as from a retained foreign body, can lead to scarring and narrowing of a bronchial lumen.

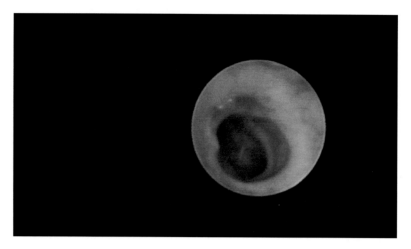

Figure 5.9 Complete bronchial rings.

- – Complete bronchial rings can be a cause of bronchial stenosis, though these are less common than complete tracheal rings.[17] This can be an extension of a segment of complete tracheal rings or a separate diagnosis. Complete bronchial rings are shown in **Figure 5.9**.
- *Bronchomalacia*, like tracheomalacia, is the dynamic collapse of the bronchi during exhalation.[19–21]
  - – As the bronchi have cartilage rings just as the trachea does, abnormalities in the bronchial cartilage can lead to collapse of the posterior bronchial wall into the lumen and can be seen on bronchoscopy, as shown in **Video 5.4**. As with tracheomalacia, this can depend on the level of anesthesia, the use of positive pressure during the procedure, and how heavily the patient is breathing.
  - – Bronchomalacia can be localized to one part of the bronchial tree or present diffusely throughout the bronchi. The mainstem bronchi are the most likely to be affected by malacia, though any bronchus can be involved.
- *Bronchial compression*, like tracheal compression, is caused by an extrinsic force on the bronchus, resulting in the narrowing of the lumen.
  - – Mass effect lesions, such as a tumor or an enlarged lymph node, can result in bronchial compression. Blood vessels and vascular rings generally affect the trachea and are less likely to cause bronchial compression.[23]
  - – Thoracic scoliosis can result in bronchial compression from the spine and blood vessels or structures due to rotation and distortion of their anatomic location.
  - – In infants and young children, there is often a mild compression of the left-sided airways due to the heart.[24]
- *Intraluminal lesions* can cause bronchial obstruction, which may lead to mucus plugging, retained secretions, and post-obstructive pneumonia.
  - – Foreign bodies typically cause acute bronchial obstruction, occurring more commonly in younger patients or children with developmental delays. Nuts and other organic material can cause significant local mucosal inflammation (**Figure 5.10** shows a piece of carrot lodged into the bronchus intermedius).
  - – Other intraluminal lesions include endobronchial tumors such as carcinoid tumors and endobronchial granulomas from infections such as tuberculosis or histoplasmosis.[25] **Figure 5.11** shows an endobronchial granuloma as a result of histoplasmosis.
- *Mucus plugging* is a common problem in children. Particularly in smaller airways, thick and sticky mucus can lead to airway obstruction with impaired mucociliary clearance and becomes difficult to remove.
  - – Whereas this more commonly occurs in segmental bronchi, it can be seen in lobar or mainstem bronchi.
  - – Mucus plugging can be secondary to an infection or related to underlying impairments in mucociliary clearance. Lack of humidification of patients, who are intubated or who have a tracheostomy, can also lead to drying of mucus and resultant plugging.

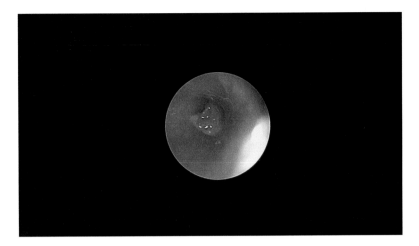

Figure 5.10 Piece of carrot lodged into the bronchus intermedius.

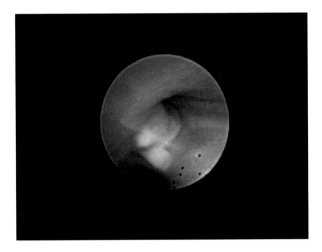

Figure 5.11 Endobronchial granuloma as a result of histoplasmosis.

- In some instances, mucus plugs cannot be removed despite direct visualization and suctioning through the flexible bronchoscope. Chapters 8 and 9 describe additional interventions and techniques that may be used.
- *Bronchitis* is a general term describing inflammation in the airways.
  - Bronchitis can encompass mucosal edema and friability, secretions in the lower airways (purulent or non-purulent), or cobblestoning/follicular appearance of the airways (examples are shown in Figure 5.12a–c).
  - Bronchitis can be diffuse or localized to a part of the airway.
  - Secretions can be from infection, aspiration, or impaired mucociliary clearance. Bronchoalveolar lavage can help identify the cause of bronchitis.
- *Pulmonary hemorrhage* is the presence of blood in the lower airway, as seen in Figure 5.13.
  - Bleeding into the lung can have a variety of causes, including trauma, infection, bronchiectasis, and pulmonary vasculitis;[27] the endoscopic management of the patient with pulmonary hemorrhage is discussed in Chapter 9.
  - If there is active, ongoing bleeding, bright red blood is visualized in the airway. Blood can arise from the pulmonary arterial circulation system (lower pressure) or the bronchial arteries (under

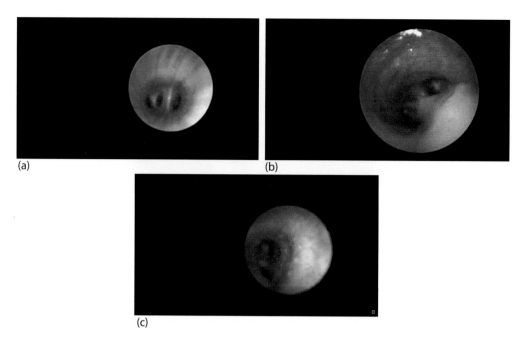

(a)　　　　　　　　　　(b)

(c)

Figure 5.12 (a–c) Bronchitis. Bronchitis can encompass mucosal edema and friability (shown in a), secretions in the lower airways (purulent or non-purulent, as seen in panel b), or cobblestoning/follicular appearance of the airways, in panel c.

Figure 5.13 Pulmonary hemorrhage.

systemic blood pressure).[28] The location of the airway bleeding may correspond to the location of the bleeding vessel, but this can be difficult to ascertain when there is massive bleeding.

-   Pulmonary opacities on chest imaging can be due to blood in the airways and should be suspected in the setting of hemoptysis and an unexplained drop in the hemoglobin content. Diffuse alveolar hemorrhage can be caused by a variety of diseases, such as in the setting of capillaritis (inflammation of small blood vessels in the lungs) or pulmonary hemosiderosis, and sequential bronchoalveolar lavage will show progressively more hemorrhagic aliquots.[2,7,28]

Video 5.4 Bronchomalacia.

PEARLS

- Bronchomalacia and tracheomalacia often occur together but can also be seen independently of one another.
- Bronchomalacia and bronchial compression can be difficult to distinguish, similar to tracheomalacia and tracheal compression. Bronchomalacia is a dynamic process and occurs during the expiratory phase of the respiratory cycle.
- The finding of granulation tissue in a bronchus should raise suspicion of a retained foreign body.
- Evaluation and management of certain lower airway pathologies, including the management of pulmonary hemorrhage and biopsies or removal of endobronchial lesions, must be performed by an experienced endoscopist, as there can be significant associated risk and complications.

CONCLUSION

Bronchoscopic evaluation of the lower airways is an important tool to help understand pulmonary disease in children. Flexible and rigid bronchoscopy can help identify both anatomic and dynamic processes in the lower airways of children. It is essential to be able to identify normal lower airway anatomy in order to be able to recognize abnormalities. As pathology can occur at any level of the lower airway, a complete evaluation is necessary to provide a comprehensive and thorough evaluation.

REFERENCES

1. Faro, A., et al., Official American Thoracic Society technical standards: flexible airway endoscopy in children. *Am J Respir Crit Care Med*, 2015. 191(9): p. 1066–80.
2. Miller, R.J., et al., Flexible bronchoscopy. *Clin Chest Med*, 2018. 39(1): p. 1–16.
3. Wood, R.E., Pediatric bronchoscopy. *Chest Surg Clin N Am*, 1996. 6(2): p. 237–51.
4. Midulla, F., et al., Flexible endoscopy of paediatric airways. *Eur Respir J*, 2003. 22(4): p. 698–708.
5. Chassagnon, G., et al., Tracheobronchial branching abnormalities: lobe-based classification scheme. *RadioGraphics*, 2016. 36(2): p. 358–73.
6. NOMENCLATURE of broncho-pulmonary anatomy; an international nomenclature accepted by the Thoracic Society. *Thorax*, 1950. 5(3): p. 222–8.
7. Chassagnon, G., et al., Tracheobronchial branching abnormalities: lobe-based classification scheme-erratum. *Radiographics*, 2016. 36(4): p. 1258.
8. Vijayasekaran, S., Pediatric airway pathology. *Frontiers in Pediatrics*, 2020. 8(246).
9. Walner, D.L., M.S. Loewen, and R.E. Kimura, Neonatal subglottic stenosis: incidence and trends. *Laryngoscope*, 2001. 111(1): p. 48–51.
10. Duynstee, M.L., et al., Subglottic stenosis after endolaryngeal intubation in infants and children: result of wound healing processes. *Int J Pediatr Otorhinolaryngol*, 2002. 62(1): p. 1–9.
11. Myer, C.M., 3rd, D.M. O'Connor, and R.T. Cotton, Proposed grading system for subglottic stenosis based on endotracheal tube sizes. *Ann Otol Rhinol Laryngol*, 1994. 103(4 Pt 1): p. 319–23.
12. Achildi, O. and H. Grewal, Congenital anomalies of the esophagus. *Otolaryngol Clin North Am*, 2007. 40(1): p. 219–44, viii.
13. Benjamin, B. and A. Inglis, Minor congenital laryngeal clefts: diagnosis and classification. *Ann Otol Rhinol Laryngol*, 1989. 98(6): p. 417–20.
14. Griffith, C. and T. Liversedge, Laryngeal clefts. *BJA Educ*, 2014. 15(5): p. 237–41.
15. Herrera, P., et al., The current state of congenital tracheal stenosis. *Pediatr Surg Int*, 2007. 23(11): p. 1033–44.
16. Rimell, F.L. and S.E. Stool, Diagnosis and management of pediatric tracheal stenosis. *Otolaryngol Clin North Am*, 1995. 28(4): p. 809–27.

17. Schweiger, C., A.P. Cohen, and M.J. Rutter, Tracheal and bronchial stenoses and other obstructive conditions. *J Thorac Dis*, 2016. 8(11): p. 3369–78.

18. Ashiku, S.K. and D.J. Mathisen, Idiopathic laryngotracheal stenosis. *Chest Surg Clin N Am*, 2003. 13(2): p. 257–69.

19. Boogaard, R., et al., Tracheomalacia and bronchomalacia in children: incidence and patient characteristics. *Chest*, 2005. 128(5): p. 3391–7.

20. Wallis, C., et al., ERS statement on tracheomalacia and bronchomalacia in children. *Eur Respir J*, 2019. 54(3).

21. Wallis, C., et al., Tracheomalacia and bronchomalacia in children: response to the ERS statement. *Eur Respir J*, 2019. 54(6).

22. Strife, J.L., A.S. Baumel, and J.S. Dunbar, Tracheal compression by the innominate artery in infancy and childhood. *Radiology*, 1981. 139(1): p. 73–5.

23. Stanger, P., R.V. Lucas, Jr., and J.E. Edwards, Anatomic factors causing respiratory distress in acyanotic congenital cardiac disease. Special reference to bronchial obstruction. *Pediatrics*, 1969. 43(5): p. 760–9.

24. Erwin, E.A., M.E. Gerber, and R.T. Cotton, Vascular compression of the airway: indications for and results of surgical management. *Int J Pediatr Otorhinolaryngol*, 1997. 40(2–3): p. 155–62.

25. Pio, L., et al., Pediatric airway tumors: a report from the international network of pediatric airway teams (INPAT). *Laryngoscope*, 2020. 130(4): p. E243–E251.

26. Lertsburapa, K., J.W. Schroeder, Jr., and C. Sullivan, Tracheal cartilaginous sleeve in patients with craniosynostosis syndromes: a meta-analysis. *J Pediatr Surg*, 2010. 45(7): p. 1438–44.

27. Leatherman, J.W., S.F. Davies, and J.R. Hoidal, Alveolar hemorrhage syndromes: diffuse microvascular lung hemorrhage in immune and idiopathic disorders. *Medicine (Baltimore)*, 1984. 63(6): p. 343–61.

28. Lara, A.R. and M.I. Schwarz, Diffuse alveolar hemorrhage. *Chest*, 2010. 137(5): p. 1164–71.

6

Upper airway bronchoscopic approach and diagnostic procedures

KARA D. MEISTER AND DON HAYES, JR.

INTRODUCTION

This chapter describes the techniques and potential complications of upper airway evaluation and intervention. For a summary of the equipment discussed in this chapter, please refer to Chapters 2 and 3. For an anatomic atlas, discussion of the normal anatomy, and discussion of common pathology of the upper airway, please refer to Chapter 4.

There are several indications for upper airway evaluation in pediatric patients, including stertor, nasal obstruction, stridor, sleep-disordered breathing or obstructive sleep apnea, dysphonia, or dysphagia. There are other indications, such as an unexplained cough or hemoptysis, which warrant a full evaluation of the airway, including upper and lower airway evaluation. Any clinical symptom or suspected pathology which requires an endoscopic view of the airways to aid in diagnosis can be considered an indication for diagnostic upper airway evaluation. This should be tempered with safety and ease of the procedures, as well as the ability of the procedures to be able to aid in diagnosis, given the clinical context of the patient.

DRUG-INDUCED SLEEP ENDOSCOPY (DISE)

PREPARATION, POSITIONING, AND ANESTHESIA

- The patient positioning should match the indication for the evaluation and clinical history as far as feasible. A small pillow without a shoulder roll is generally preferred for DISE.
- The endoscopist should stand wherever is most comfortable and practiced, either to the patient's side or from the head of the bed. Access to definitely control the patient's airway in case of emergency should be maintained.
- Video monitors should be easily seen, for both the endoscopic projection and the vital signs.
- Anesthesia for sleep endoscopy is controversial and the choice depends on the ability of the agent to be titrated to achieve the most representative sleep state. Deeper levels of sedation are associated with

DOI: 10.1201/9781003106234-6

decreased muscle tone, airway collapsibility, and tendency toward atelectasis. A discussion between the anesthesiologist and the endoscopist about the anesthetic agents and administration techniques should be held prior to the patient being sedated.[1] Documentation of the anesthetic choices in the operative report is helpful.

- Nasal, oral, or "blow-by" oxygen are sometimes employed. An oral airway connected *via* an endotracheal tube (ETT) adaptor can be helpful (**Figure 6.1**), but it should be removed as tolerated so not to alter the anatomic findings. A nasal airway should be avoided until the upper airway has been fully evaluated as passage of a nasal airway can cause edema, epistaxis, and potentially laryngospasm.
- The environment should mimic a sleep state: dimmed lights, low noise, and comfortable room temperature.
- The polysomnogram should be reviewed, and the SpO_2 nadir and CO_2 data should be noted, with these providing soft limits during the procedure.[2]

EQUIPMENT

- DISE can be performed with either a flexible laryngoscope or a flexible bronchoscope. Using the smallest diameter tool possible will have potentially less impact on resistance and discomfort, and will afford the most reliable examination.
- Advantages of a flexible bronchoscope are the ability to provide oxygen *via* insufflation, to suction excess secretions, apply topical lidocaine to the larynx, and proceed continuously with lower airway bronchoscopic evaluation.
- Advantages of a flexible laryngoscope are the availability of sizes down to 2.5 mm, potentially better ergonomics for the proceduralist, and less costly instrument processing.

TECHNIQUE

- The examination begins with inspection of the patient. The patient should be in a sleep-like state, preferably snoring as a result of obstructions (if obstructions are included in the clinical history), with natural positioning. The patient's overall habitus, jaw position, neck anatomy and hyoid position, chest wall anatomy, and chest movement should be examined. It may be helpful to obtain photo documentation of pertinent findings, such as retrognathia or an abnormal bite.

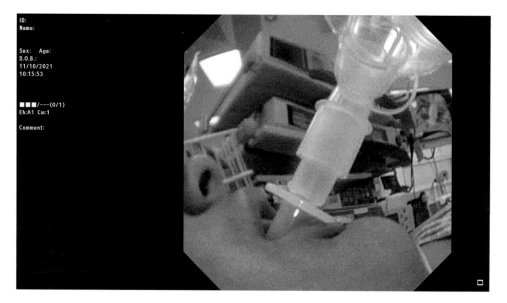

Figure 6.1 An oral airway is connected to the adaptor of an endotracheal tube, which is connected to the ventilator circuit.

- Each side of the nasal airway should be evaluated, with careful attention to the internal nasal valve. The nasal valve area is formed by the nasal septum, the caudal border of the upper lateral cartilage, the head of the inferior turbinate, and the pyriform aperture; it is also marked by the transition of skin to respiratory epithelium. Photo documentation of each side of the anterior nose and the size of the inferior turbinates is helpful; note whether the patient received nasal decongestant as this can alter findings of nasal obstruction.
- The scope is passed through the nasal cavity. The middle meatus is generally preferred as it is often larger than the nasal floor, affords a more subtle angle for the scope to pass the nasopharynx, and is good practice for transnasal fiber-optic intubation. Any septal deformity or obstructing lesion preventing passage of the scope should be noted.
- At the nasopharynx, any lesions or stenosis should be described, and the degree of adenoid obstruction and retropalatal collapse should be documented.
- At the oropharynx, the anatomy and dynamic configurations of the velum, retropalatal space, uvula, and lateral pharyngeal walls should be described. Size of the palatine tonsils and the degree (none, partial, complete) and pattern (circular, anterior-posterior, mixed, etc.) of collapse at the level of the tonsils is described. The tongue is evaluated for macroglossia, glossoptosis, or hypertrophy of the lingual tonsils.
- The examination should be dynamic, with movement of the scope proximal and distal throughout the respiratory cycle to get a comprehensive account of how the structures and tissues interact during different phases of the respiratory cycle, and with different maneuvers such as light jaw thrust or head turn.
- In infants and children, attention is also directed at the supraglottic larynx for evidence of laryngomalacia, epiglottic prolapse, and active reflux.

DOCUMENTATION

- There are a number of classification schemes, and, until a consensus is reached, the endoscopist should chose a classification system that is easily reproduced for consistency.[3–5]
- Systematic photo documentation in the operative report is strongly encouraged.
- Video recording of examinations is beneficial for referring back to at subsequent appointments, for multidisciplinary collaboration, and for educating parents and trainees (see Videos 6.1–6.4).

Video 6.1 A patient is prepared for sleep endoscopy using an oral airway connected to the ventilator circuit *via* an ETT adaptor. Note that the oral airway is removed to start the examination.

Video 6.2 Sleep endoscopy, examining the nasal airway, nasopharynx, and oropharynx.

Video 6.3 Sleep endoscopy, examining the retrolingual space, hypopharynx, and supraglottic larynx. Note the laryngomalacia evidenced by prolapsing of the arytenoid cartilages.

Video 6.4 Sleep endoscopy, illustrating glossoptosis and hypertrophy of the lingual tonsils. This is best evaluated once the oral airway is removed.

COMPLICATIONS AND DISPOSITION

- Epistaxis
- Laryngospasm/bronchospasm
- Oxyhemoglobin desaturations
- Atelectasis
- Most patients can be discharged on the same day following recovery in the post-anesthesia care unit

PEARLS

- The best examination mimics the clinical history. The patient should be permitted to snore and obstruct within the confines of safety. Positioning and sedation may need to be dynamic to recreate the clinical history, such as employing a head turn or lightening the anesthesia until snoring and obstructions are appreciated, as to meet the goal of the examination: guiding treatment recommendations.

BRONCHOSCOPE-ASSISTED TRANSNASAL INTUBATION

Transnasal intubation can be facilitated by use of a flexible bronchoscope while allowing evaluation of upper airway anatomy and mechanics.

TEAM PREPARATION

- There are several nuances to this technique, and we describe our preferences with the understanding that the best approach is that with which the team performing the procedure is most comfortable.
- A bronchoscopist, first assistant, anesthesiologist, circulating nurse, and, if possible, a surgical technician and anesthesia assistant should be available to discuss the plan.

PATIENT PREPARATION

- Full-face nebulization of lidocaine and racemic epinephrine can facilitate anesthesia management.
- In some patients, topical anesthesia of the nose with additional lidocaine and topical decongestant *via* cotton pledgets can also be helpful; in other children, however, this will cause agitation and may hinder cooperation with the procedure.
- Glycopyrrolate may be considered for secretion management.

EQUIPMENT

- An extended length endotracheal tube (ETT) will likely be required. This can be either a nasal right-angle endotracheal (RAE) tube, a microlaryngoscopy tube (MLT, standard internal diameter [available in 4.0 mm, 5.0 mm and 6.0 mm] with increased length) or two ETTs fashioned together for extra length. In small children, a standard 3.5 or 4.0 micro-cuffed ETT may be long enough, with the advantage of the micro-cuff being easier to traverse the nasal cavity than a standard cuff.
- The tube should be warmed in saline, to make it more malleable, and connected to an adapter, such as the Bodai BRONCH-SAFE airway connector, prior to loading on the bronchoscope.
- If a 3.5 ETT is being used with a 3.1-mm OD bronchoscope (such as the Olympus BF-XP190), the ETT connector should be upsized to a 4.0 ETT connector.
- The ETT and connector should be loaded at the most proximal aspect of the bronchoscope; the diaphragm of the Bodai BRONCH-SAFE airway connector will hug the proximal aspect of the bronchoscope.
- Oxygen tubing is connected to the suction port of the bronchoscope and set to 1–2 L/min of insufflation (**Figure 6.2**).
- Two suctions should be available, turned on, and able to reach the field without tension: one for oral secretions, and one to attach to the bronchoscope, if needed.
- Topical lidocaine with a few milliliters of air should be drawn into a slip-tip syringe and properly labeled.

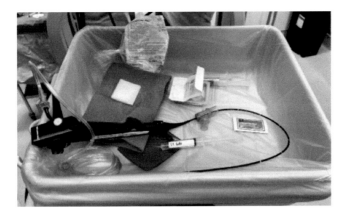

Figure 6.2 The Bodai BRONCH-SAFE™ connector, oxygen tubing, and lidocaine are prepared for transnasal fiber-optic intubation.

- Dry gauze should be available for the bronchoscopist, as well as for the assistant.
- The ETT and bronchoscope should be well lubricated, and easy passage of the scope through the ETT should be confirmed by rehearsal.
- It is our practice to have a full airway emergency cart in the room, which includes various devices such as laryngeal mask airways (LMAs), rigid ventilating bronchoscopes, and a tracheostomy tray.

POSITIONING

- The patient should be maintained in an upright position as tolerated, preferably with gentle jaw thrust provided by the assistant. In some situations, an assistant manually pulling the patient's tongue forward can be helpful.
- The bronchoscopist should stand at either the side or at the head of the bed, depending on personal experience and comfort, with easy visualization of the bronchoscopy feed and the vital signs.
- The assistant should be able to reach the oral suction and the ETT and should have a video screen of the bronchoscopy image in their field of view.
- The anesthesiologist should be at the head of the bed, with access to both screens, the ventilator, emergency supplies, and medications. It is sometimes helpful to have a second anesthesia provider with access to the IV and to provide assistance in emergency situations.

TECHNIQUE

- It is our practice to insert the bronchoscope into the nose rather than first inserting a nasal airway or the ETT as these extra procedures risk trauma and epistaxis and hinder the maneuverability of the bronchoscope.
- Begin by defogging the lens of the bronchoscope.
- Once in the nose, the path through the middle meatus provides the gentlest curve around the palate and can best facilitate passage of the ETT.
- If there are redundant soft tissues, insufflation of oxygen can be used to distract these tissues and improve visualization.
- Gentle jaw thrust, or even grasping the patient's anterior tongue with forward traction, can also facilitate a view of the larynx.
- Once the larynx is in view, topical lidocaine can be administered *via* the biopsy valve. In addition, supplemental oxygen can be provided *via* the suction valve.
- The bronchoscope is advanced into the trachea by aiming toward the anterior commissure of the larynx, and then employing downward flexion while traversing the glottis.
- Once tracheal rings are visualized, the bronchoscope is advanced to the carina.

- The bronchoscopist should diligently maintain a view of the carina at all times. It is usually best to have an assistant pass the ETT while the bronchoscopist keeps focus on the carina, providing gentle insufflation of oxygen into the trachea *via* the bronchoscope.
- Passage of the ETT is facilitated by rotation and gentle pressure, and adequate lubrication. If resistance is met, slight withdrawal and counterclockwise rotation can promote passage.
- Once the ETT is in the trachea, the ventilator circuit is connected to the Bodai BRONCH-SAFE™ airway connector. The oxygen is switched to suction, and any secretions can be cleared. Proper positioning of the ETT above the carina is confirmed, and the bronchoscope is then withdrawn with care not to withdraw the ETT concurrently.

PEARLS

- Choice of the bronchoscope and ETT should be guided by the patient's age, size, and anatomy. In general, the bronchoscope should pass easily through the ETT but without excess room as too much space can allow for tissue to be caught between and hinder maneuverability. Some authors also advocate for the use of a Parker Flex-Tip™ ETT because the curved tip of the tube more closely hugs the bronchoscope.

INTUBATION *VIA* A SUPRAGLOTTIC AIRWAY DEVICE

If transnasal intubation is not feasible, consideration for intubation *via* a supraglottic airway device (SGA), such as a classic laryngeal mask airway (LMA) or air-Q, should be considered. This is especially useful in infants with micrognathia, such as Pierre Robin sequence, in which direct laryngoscopy is difficult.

EQUIPMENT

- The key to successful intubation *via* an SGA is to rehearse the mechanics of the equipment completely prior to beginning the procedure.
- A classic LMA has two limitations to being a conduit for endotracheal intubation. First, the length of the LMA is such that two endotracheal tubes (one ETT to be positioned endotracheally, and one ETT as a pusher tube) are needed to traverse the length of the LMA. Second, the aperture bars must be removed to allow passage of the ETT. If a cuffed endotracheal tube is used, the airway connector of the ETT cannot be used, and it is imperative to practice full passage of the ETTs, the pilot balloon, and the LMA prior to beginning the procedure.
- The air-Q intubating laryngeal airway is designed to overcome some of the barriers of a classic LMA, including a shorter and wider shaft, lack of aperture bars, and removable 15 mm circuit adapters.

TECHNIQUE

- Once the LMA or air-Q is in position, the technique for intubation is similar to transnasal intubation.
- Removal of the SGA over the endotracheal tube is recommended once the endotracheal tube is confirmed to be in the airway.
- The ETT adapter must be removed, and the ETT must be stabilized (by forceps, the flexible bronchoscope, or an airway exchange catheter) during removal of the SGA. If a second, "pusher" ETT is used, it is grasped with pediatric Magill forceps or by an assistant and stabilized as the LMA is withdrawn. The second ETT is then cut as needed to eliminate dead space, and the ETT connector and ventilation circuit are connected.[6]
- Sufficient lubrication of the bronchoscope, the SGA, and the ETT is key to a successful intubation.

CONCLUSION

Performing an evaluation of the upper airway requires clinical expertise, procedural skill, and a safe environment with proper equipment and support. Sleep endoscopy in children can be performed by either pulmonologists or otolaryngologists and is an important diagnostic tool for evaluation of the upper airway. Bronchoscopists should be ready to employ endoscopic guidance to aid in difficult intubations, such as transnasal fiber-optic intubation or intubation *via* a supraglottic airway device.

TIPS FOR CLINICAL PRACTICE

- Using the smallest scope possible may be advantageous in performing pediatric sleep endoscopy so as to minimize alterations in nasal airflow and to decrease patient stimulation.
- Rehearsing the steps of fiber-optic intubation is key to ensuring that the ETTs, scopes, and other equipment are of compatible sizes.
- If there is resistance to maneuvering the ETT during a fiber-optic intubation, disconnecting the ETT (or Bodai adaptor) from the circuit temporarily can help facilitate mobility.

REFERENCES

1. Charakorn N, Kezirian EJ. Drug-induced sleep endoscopy. *Otolaryngol Clin North Am.* 2016 Dec;49(6):1359–72.
2. Adler AC, Musso MF, Mehta DK, Chandrakantan A. Pediatric drug induced sleep endoscopy: A simple sedation recipe. *Ann Otol Rhinol Laryngol.* 2020 May;129(5):428–33.
3. Williamson A, Ibrahim SR, Coutras SW, Carr MM. Pediatric drug-induced sleep endoscopy: Technique and scoring system. *Cureus [Internet].* 2020 Oct 2 [cited 2021 Jan 2]; Available from: https://www.cureus.com/articles/41034-pediatric-drug-induced-sleep-endoscopy-technique-and-scoring-system
4. Wilcox LJ, Bergeron M, Reghunathan S, Ishman SL. An updated review of pediatric drug-induced sleep endoscopy: Review of pediatric drug-induced sleep endoscopy. *Laryngoscope Investig Otolaryngol.* 2017 Dec;2(6):423–31.
5. Friedman NR, Parikh SR, Ishman SL, Ruiz AG, El-Hakim H, Ulualp SO, et al. The current state of pediatric drug-induced sleep endoscopy: The current state of pediatric DISE. *Laryngoscope.* 2017 Jan;127(1):266–72.
6. Lauder GR, Thomas M, Ungern-Sternberg BS von, Engelhardt T. Volatiles or TIVA: Which is the standard of care for pediatric airway procedures? A pro-con discussion. *Pediatr Anesth.* 2020;30(3):209–20.

7

Lower airway bronchoscopic approach and diagnostic procedures

BRANDY JOHNSON, STEPHEN FRANKLIN, AND MAUREEN JOSEPHSON

INTRODUCTION

Evaluation of the lower airway provides valuable information for the management of children experiencing persistent pulmonary symptoms, recurrent lower airway infections, or acute changes in respiratory status. Bronchoscopy is often approached in these instances when medical intervention has not been impactful or timely diagnosis is required. Either rigid or flexible bronchoscopy can be utilized for the evaluation of the lower airways; however, the branching configuration of the lower bronchial tree precludes routine use of the rigid bronchoscope distal to the segmental bronchi. Please reference Chapter 5 for a detailed review of the tracheobronchial anatomy.

Each type of bronchoscopy offers distinct advantages when used for evaluating lower airway disorders. Rigid bronchoscopy allows the operator to secure the airway, provide ventilation through the endoscope, and introduce instruments through a large working channel. The use of the rigid bronchoscope is preferred when clinicians are faced with evaluating the upper and proximal lower airway anatomy, pulmonary hemorrhage, or suspected foreign body aspiration. Additional therapeutic indications include the need for deep tissue biopsy, airway dilation, stent placement, laser therapy, and debulking of proximal airway tumors. On

Table 7.1 Indications for bronchoscopic evaluation of the lower airways in pediatric patients

- Anatomical evaluation
- Persistent respiratory symptoms (i.e., chronic cough, wheeze, stridor, hemoptysis, apnea, cyanosis)
- Infectious/inflammatory concerns
- Abnormal radiologic findings (i.e., atelectasis, ground glass or tree-in-bud opacities, pulmonary nodules)
- Tissue sampling (i.e., endobronchial or transbronchial biopsy)
- Examination of artificial airway
- Therapeutic intervention (i.e., alleviate airway obstruction, achieve hemorrhage control, foreign body removal, stent placement)

the other hand, flexible endoscopes allow bronchoscopists to perform a complete evaluation of the tracheo-bronchial tree to the quaternary subdivision, including a dynamic assessment. Flexible bronchoscopy also enables intervention on distal airway pathology, as well as sampling of the alveolar contents for infectious analysis. Despite these differing applications, it should be recognized that the two types of bronchoscopy can be performed in combination to evaluate the lower airways, where necessary. The bronchoscopic approach taken will be dictated, not only by the suspected pathology, but also by institutional resources and operator experience.

Surgical and pulmonary teams frequently collaborate intra-operatively during lower airway evaluations. Pre-operative consultation with a multi-disciplinary airway team helps to maximize resources available when surgical interventions are anticipated. During the performance of the procedure, there is interdisciplinary communication between the anesthesia team and bronchoscopy team throughout the evaluation and management process while the bronchoscopy is being performed.

INDICATIONS FOR LOWER AIRWAY EVALUATION

- Flexible bronchoscopy allows clinicians to perform diagnostic and therapeutic interventions in evaluating the lower airways and lung parenchyma of patients presenting with chronic respiratory symptoms or abnormal radiologic findings (Table 7.1) (see Chapter 2).
- Rigid and flexible approaches together are the mainstay of lower airway endoscopy; however, flexible bronchoscopy will be the focus of this chapter, given its unique procedural capabilities within the distal airways.
- Sampling superficial mucosa, abnormal lesions, and mucus of the lower airways provides a basis for analyzing the cellular content and tissue structure when evaluating for inflammation, infection, malignancy, or abnormal architecture.
- Multiple investigative techniques are performed through the flexible endoscope, such as bronchial brushings, bronchial washing, bronchoalveolar lavage (BAL), and endobronchial and transbronchial biopsies.
- Flexible bronchoscopy also serves as a conduit for specialized therapeutic procedures in the setting of airway stenosis, tumors, persistent air leaks, and foreign body removal.

POTENTIAL COMPLICATIONS

Lower airway bronchoscopy is usually well tolerated; however, risks of the procedure and anesthesia must be considered for every patient, especially those with acute clinical presentations or high-risk co-morbidities. Potential complications should be discussed with the patient and parents/guardian during the consent process. No absolute contraindications exist for lower airway bronchoscopy. Relative contraindications are cardiovascular instability, uncontrolled coagulopathy or bleeding diathesis, refractory hypoxemia, and severe bronchospasm.

- Minor consequences include:
  - Transient hypoxemia and hypercapnia
  - Cough
  - Fever
  - Bleeding
  - Iatrogenic edema
- More serious complications are rare, with the risk of occurrence increasing in the face of advanced diagnostic and interventional techniques; these include:
  - Respiratory failure
  - Significant hemorrhage
  - Airway trauma
  - Pneumothorax
  - Bronchospasm
  - Nosocomial infection
  - Intra-pulmonary spread of infection

EQUIPMENT

For a full review of equipment required for performing rigid and flexible bronchoscopy, please see Chapter 2. Many pieces of equipment are standard across bronchoscopy procedures, although specialized techniques warrant unique instruments for tissue retrieval and preservation. Suggested tools pertinent to lower airway bronchoscopy and routine diagnostic evaluation are outlined in **Table 7.2** and are included in **Figure 7.1**. The tools and approach may vary among bronchoscopists and hospitals.

Table 7.2 List of recommended equipment for bronchoscopy of the lower airway

Informed consent with patient identifiers	Lidocaine solution (1% and 2% concentrations)
Cardiopulmonary monitoring	Sterile saline, warmed to body temperature (37°C)
Face masks, eye protection, surgical gowns, and assortment of gloves (non-sterile, sterile)	Slip-tip syringes

Bronchoscopy cart
  Light source
  Video monitor
  Image processor
	Specimen traps

Flexible bronchoscopes, two sizes recommended
  Sizes: outer diameter 2.2–6.3 mm, inner channel 1.2–3.2 mm
	Optional tools
	  Rigid bronchoscopes
	  Ventilation devices
	  Connection for supplemental oxygen
	  Endotracheal tube adapter

Suction apparatus	Gauze sponges
Anti-fog solution	Transbronchial aspiration needles
Bronchoscope lubricant	Cytology brushes
	Biopsy forceps
	Fixative solution (i.e., 10% formalin, glutaraldehyde)
	Fluoroscopy

Note: Supplies will vary based on provider preference. Specialized tools for endobronchial ultrasound-guided procedures and navigational bronchoscopy are discussed in Chapter 8.

Bronchoscope Cart
1. Video monitor
2. Image processor
3. Light source
4. Bronchoscope lubricant
5. Lidocaine solution
6. Sterile saline
7. Specimen trap
8. Slip tip syringes
9. Anti-fog solution
10. Ventilation pressure keep
11. Sterile specimen containers

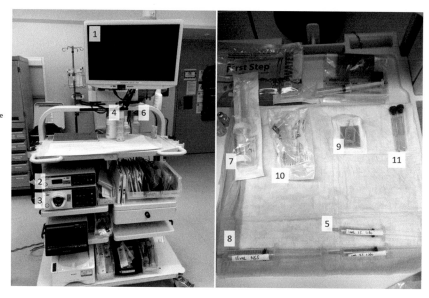

Figure 7.1 Bronchoscopy cart with standard supplies for conducting an anatomical evaluation of the lower airways and bronchoalveolar lavage.

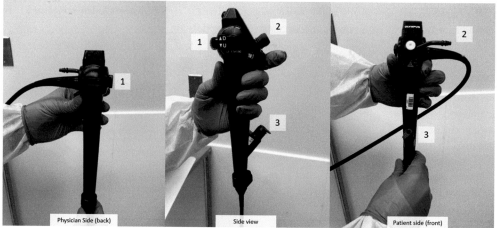

1. Extension/Flexion control of working tip
2. Suction control/port
3. Suction Channel/Working channel

Figure 7.2 Olympus® Diagnostic Bronchoscope (BF-1TH190) with 4.0-mm external diameter and 2.8-mm working channel.

- Multiple endoscopes of differing sizes should be readily available for use during lower airway evaluations. In the event of unforeseen technical or procedural complications, providers should be able to alternate bronchoscopes (**Figures 7.2–7.4**).
- In cases that may warrant therapeutic intervention, proceduralists should consider having rigid bronchoscopes and related accessories prepared. If not trained to perform rigid bronchoscopy, the primary evaluating team should give advance notice to operators comfortable with the use of rigid instruments that their involvement in the case could be necessary.
- Lidocaine is used for topical anesthesia, when the neuromuscular blockade is not present, to prevent reflex activation of the airways during mechanical stimulation. Preparations containing 1% or 2% solution are applied to the larynx and carina. Although there is no established consensus on maximal

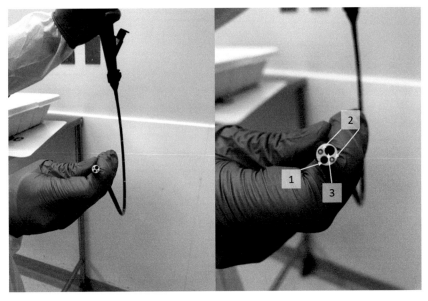

1. Objective lens
2. Light source
3. Suction Channel/Working channel

Figure 7.3 End-on view of the Olympus Diagnostic Bronchoscope (BF-1TH190).

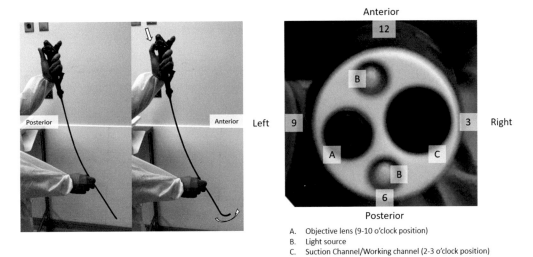

A. Objective lens (9-10 o'clock position)
B. Light source
C. Suction Channel/Working channel (2-3 o'clock position)

Figure 7.4 Detailed view of the Olympus Diagnostic Bronchoscope (BF-1TH190) from the end-on vantage point and demonstration of flexed positioning.

dosing, application of 4 milligrams lidocaine per kilogram bodyweight to the airway has been determined to be safe in pediatric patients, despite elevated drug plasma levels occasionally being detected at this topical dose. Some practitioners will use higher total doses of lidocaine when administered as multiple individual boluses across a prolonged period. Topical lidocaine doses of 7–8.5 milligrams per kilogram have been proven to be safe when delivered as smaller boluses repeatedly over 45 minutes. It is recommended that providers consider clinical factors that would predispose the patient to local anesthetic toxicity and modify the dose accordingly.

- Saline aliquots can be defined as fixed volumes or volumes adjusted for bodyweight. See Chapter 2 for additional details.

GENERAL PREPARATION

POSITIONING

- Patient position depends on the route of endoscopy and the patient pathology. Typically, supine positioning with the head in either a neutral or slightly extended position is preferred.
- Standing at the head of the patient allows for the most comfortable provider position during endoscopy. When standing at the right or left side of the patient's head, the bronchoscope can be aligned more naturally with the right or left mainstem bronchus, respectively.
- Video/visual monitors should be positioned on either side of the bed, or at the end of the bed, to prevent discomfort to the endoscopist.

LOWER AIRWAY INTERVENTIONS

Pre-operative planning is essential to ensure that the goals of the evaluation are met. Proceduralists should start with devising a broad differential, in the context of the clinical presentation, so that all necessary testing is ordered prior to sample processing. Review of chest imaging performed in advance of the endoscopy can provide an insight into affected regions of the airways or parenchyma and allow for a targeted evaluation and sample collection, such as in the case of persistent atelectasis, undifferentiated pulmonary infiltrates, or lung nodules. Collaboration with airway and interventional bronchoscopy experts, when available, is useful to discuss the ideal procedural approach and anticipate intra-operative complications. Lastly, communicating this plan to the anesthesia team will help all providers involved in the procedure to achieve a safe but thorough evaluation.

BRONCHOALVEOLAR LAVAGE (BAL)

- Sampling of the liquid lining the distal airways and alveoli, referred to as epithelial lining fluid, is performed through a procedure called BAL (Video 7.1).
- BAL aids in the removal of airway debris and allows for cytopathology and microbiology evaluation of samples.
- BAL fluid analysis provides insight into both infectious and non-infectious processes that cause lower airway inflammation. Non-infectious conditions that can be diagnosed through lavage analysis include alveolar proteinosis, alveolar hemorrhage, and pulmonary histiocytosis.
- Non-bronchoscopic (NB-BAL) and bronchoscopic techniques exist for performing BAL.
- NB-BAL involves instillation and retrieval of saline into the distal airways through a balloon wedge pressure catheter and suction apparatus. This technique has been demonstrated to recover adequate alveolar samples in patients with artificial airways too small to accommodate flexible bronchoscopes.
- Given the ability to directly sample a desired subsegment of the lung through visualization, bronchoscopic BAL is preferred in patients with airways large enough for the passage of bronchoscopes with a suction channel.
- There is no standard protocol that dictates the ideal volume of saline that should be used during pediatric BAL. Rather, the volume frequently varies per practitioner, with some clinicians using fixed volumes of saline for all patients, whereas others adjust to functional residual capacity and bodyweight.
- Ratjen et al. found that lavage volume adjustments for bodyweight yielded constant fractions of epithelial lining fluid in children aged 3–15 years without pulmonary disease.[19] Investigators utilized three individual aliquots of saline at one milliliter per kilogram for children weighing less than 20 kilograms and a total of a 20-milliliter aliquot, up to a total volume of three milliliters per kilogram in children weighing more than 20 kilograms.

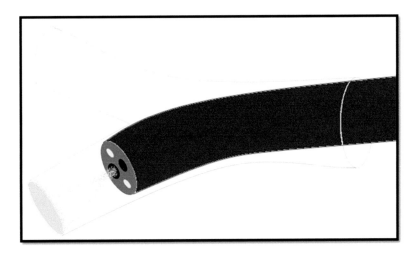

Figure 7.5 For targeted sampling during the bronchoalveolar lavage, the flexible endoscope should be wedged in the preferred subsegmental bronchus prior to instilling normal saline into the distal airways.

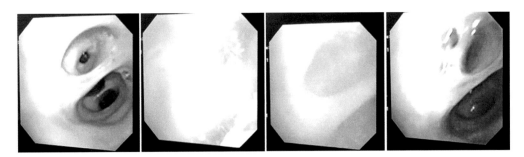

Figure 7.6 Images obtained during bronchoalveolar lavage, performed at a subsegment of the right lower lobe.

- The bronchoscopist typically selects the desired lung subsegment for instillation of sterile saline based on radiographic and endoscopic findings. The right middle lobe and lingula are preferred in diffuse disease, as these areas typically offer a maximal fluid return for BAL sampling.
- To isolate a targeted region of the lung, the bronchoscope should be wedged into the sub-bronchus of interest, while avoiding occlusion of the instrument channel (Figure 7.5).
- Instillation and recovery of lavage fluid occurs through the endoscope suction channel. There is no consensus surrounding the dwell time of lavage fluid, with many bronchoscopists not performing a dwell time. Gentle manual suction or mechanical aspiration can be used for the collection of the lavage sample into a suction trap for processing (Figure 7.6).
- Lavage acceptability is considered when fluid recovery exceeds 40% of that instilled, and few epithelial cells are noted.
- BAL fluid analysis includes the assessment of cellular and soluble components, as well as testing for the presence of microorganisms through Gram stain, culture, immunoassay, and molecular methods. See Chapter 2 for more details regarding diagnostic testing.
- The initial lavage sample is most reflective of bronchial origin and dependent on the procedure goals and can be analyzed separately or pooled with remaining lavage samples for testing.
- Microbiological studies should be performed on unfiltered BAL samples.
- Specialized infectious testing can be pursued when immunocompromised hosts are suspected of having opportunistic pathogens.

Video 7.1 Technique for performing bronchoalveolar lavage.

BRONCHIAL WASHING

- Bronchial washing involves the use of saline to clear secretions from the large airways.
- While bronchial washing can be used for the diagnosis of infection, the true application for infectious testing is controversial, given the potential for sample contamination with non-pathogenic large airway respiratory flora.
- This technique is not typically performed in isolation. Rather, bronchial washing has been used to augment cytology analysis from bronchial brushings and tissue biopsies for the investigation of endobronchial tumors in adults.
- To perform a bronchial washing, the bronchoscope does not require distal airway wedging and the volume of saline used is less than that for BAL.
- Once the instilled saline has been collected, samples are submitted for cytological and microbiological analysis.

BRONCHOSCOPIC BIOPSIES

The utilization of bronchoscopy for biopsy of the lower airway and/or pulmonary parenchyma is dependent upon the location, size, and suspected pathology. The primary approaches for bronchoscopic biopsies are cytologic brush, endobronchial, or transbronchial sampling. The latter modality can utilize image guidance to improve diagnostic yield and mitigate complications, whereas both cytologic and endobronchial biopsies are easily performed by direct visualization. The use of fine-needle aspirate or forceps can be used for transbronchial biopsies.

CYTOLOGIC BRONCHIAL BRUSHING

Cytologic brush biopsy is an easy, minimally invasive method of obtaining airway epithelial cells to assess for an assortment of pathologies (**Video 7.2**). The use of electron microscopy allows for structural analysis of cilia that can aid in the diagnosis of primary ciliary dyskinesia (PCD). Cultures and immunohistochemistry staining aid in the assessment of infection or inflammation.

Video 7.2 Technique for performing ciliary brush biopsy.

EQUIPMENT

- Cytology brush sized for the bronchoscope working channel (**Figure 7.7**).
- Glutaraldehyde solution for specimen preservation and processing. Sterile normal saline would be used for culture processing.

TECHNIQUE

1. Using a slip-tip syringe, anesthetize the carina with approximately 1–5 milligrams lidocaine per kilogram bodyweight *via* the working channel (maximum dose 300 milligrams).
2. Carefully clear any airway secretions at the level of the left and right mainstem bronchi.

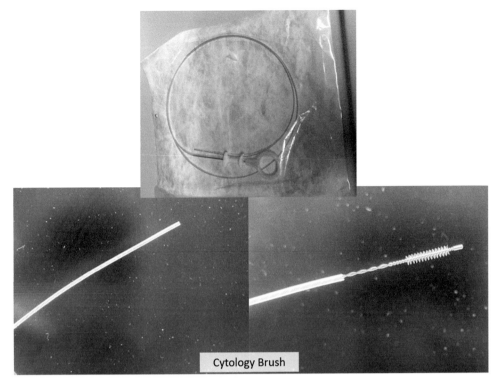

Figure 7.7 Olympus BC-204D cytology brush, working length 1150 mm, used for mucosal sampling.

3. Consider clearing the working channel by removing the bronchoscope and suctioning a small amount of normal saline through the suction port of the bronchoscope to prevent the re-introduction of airway secretions when the cytology brush is advanced through the channel.

4. Align the tip of the bronchoscope in the center of the trachea, away from the airway walls. This allows a safe distance from the bronchial mucosa so that the brush can be visualized upon introduction.

5. Before introducing the brush and guide sheath into the working channel, assess the proper deployment of the brush (Figure 7.7).

6. Introduce the cytology brush with the covering guide sheath through the working channel slowly and smoothly, keeping a careful watch on the bronchoscope tip on the video monitor.

7. Continue to advance the brush until the distal tip of the guide sheath has been passed completely through the bronchoscope.

8. Deploy the brush 1–2 centimeters distal to the guide sheath tip so that the full bristle/brush head is visualized.

9. Advance the scope so that the brush makes firm parallel contact with the medial wall of either the left or right mainstem bronchus.

10. Oscillate the brush against the bronchus, using distal to proximal thrusts for collection of cilia from the bronchial mucosa. This maneuver can be done using the bronchoscope for the oscillation fulcrum or the end of the brush wire coming from the working channel.

11. Do not retract the brush back through the working channel. Rather, carefully remove the entire bronchoscope from the airway with the brush and guide sheath still extended through the working channel. Take special note not to rub the brush head against the more proximal airways, endotracheal tube, or laryngeal mask airway. This prevents cellular structure disruption that could be caused when retracting through the working channel.

12. Once the entire scope is removed, cut the end of the ciliary brush for collection, and place the apparatus in the specimen container.
13. Repeat steps 2–10 at the opposing mainstem bronchus with a new cytology brush.

SAMPLE/SPECIMEN PROCESSING

- Preservation of the ciliary architecture is important for a detailed and accurate analysis. For cytologic evaluation, samples should be placed in a sterile container of glutaraldehyde or 10% formalin solution; however, processing is dependent upon institutional and laboratory protocols.
- For culture processing, place the sample in a container with a small amount of normal saline or against a damp Telfa pad.
- When sampling cilia for PCD, the container of glutaraldehyde should be covered in ice for transport to the laboratory.

POTENTIAL COMPLICATIONS

- Hemorrhage
- Oxyhemoglobin desaturations
- Infection

PEARLS

- Depending on the depth of sedation and the presence of neuromuscular blockade, the use of lidocaine can be omitted.
- Discuss sample processing with the pathology team, prior to collection, so that laboratory policies for appropriate biopsy handling are followed.

ENDOBRONCHIAL BIOPSY

Endobronchial biopsy is a diagnostic procedure to investigate airway structure that includes the epithelium, basement membrane, and lamina propria. Typically, this is performed for the evaluation of proximal airway tumors or mucosal abnormalities; additional indications are severe, uncontrolled asthma and sarcoidosis. Endobronchial biopsy is performed under direct visualization with the use of flexible biopsy forceps (**Figure 7.8**). For additional description of endobronchial biopsy, including the use of rigid bronchoscopy, please refer to Chapter 8.

INDICATIONS

- Endobronchial mass/lesion
- Severe, uncontrolled asthma
- Sarcoidosis

EQUIPMENT

- Reusable or disposable biopsy forceps (**Figure 7.9**)
  - The size of forceps is dependent on the working channel of the bronchoscope

TECHNIQUE

1. Inspect both proximal and distal biopsy sites, if possible. This requires the careful clearance of airway secretions to allow the best visualization of the bronchial mucosa. Avoid any pulsatile or vascular lesions.
2. Consider clearing the working channel by removing the bronchoscope from the airway and suctioning a small amount of normal saline through the suction port of the bronchoscope to prevent re-introduction of airway secretions when the biopsy forceps are advanced through the channel.

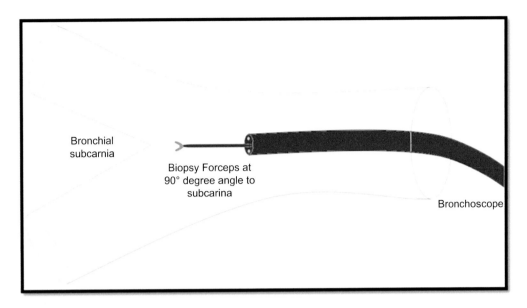

Figure 7.8 Demonstration of the perpendicular orientation of biopsy forceps relative to a subcarina for endo-bronchial biopsy.

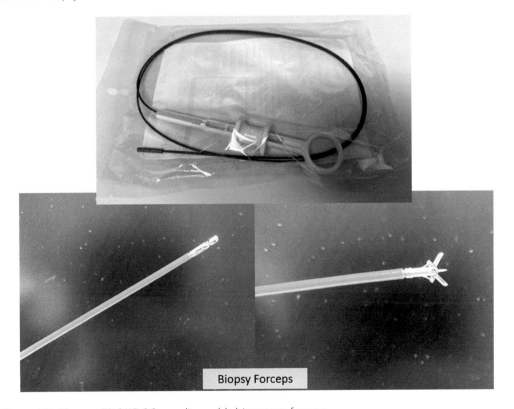

Figure 7.9 Olympus FB-241D 2.0-mm disposable biopsy cup forceps.

3. Confirm the proper open/close function of the forceps prior to introducing the instrument into the working channel of the bronchoscope.
4. Align the tip of the bronchoscope in the center of a proximal airway, away from the airway walls. This allows a safe distance from the bronchial mucosa so the forceps can be visualized upon introduction.

5. Introduce the biopsy forceps through the working channel slowly and smoothly, keeping a careful watch on the bronchoscope tip on the video monitor.

6. An assistant should help to open and close the forceps throughout the procedure. Once the distal tip of the forceps is fully introduced and can be visualized by the bronchoscope camera, re-confirm proper open/close function of the device.

7. When performing a biopsy, angle the open mouth perpendicular, or at a 90-degree angle, to the chosen subcarina, lesion, or mass (**Figure 7.8**).

COMPLICATIONS

- Hemorrhage
- Bronchospasm
- Oxyhemoglobin desaturations
- Infection

SAMPLE/SPECIMEN PROCESSING

- Samples should be placed in a sterile container of fixative, which is usually 10% formalin solution; however, processing protocols may differ, according to the institution.

TRANSBRONCHIAL BIOPSY

Transbronchial lung biopsy (TBB) through a flexible bronchoscope is a safe and minimally invasive method for obtaining peripheral lung tissue in both adults and children. The decision for obtaining a TBB is based upon accessibility to the area of biopsy interest. Newer navigational, image-guided, and virtual techniques can increase the diagnostic return and allow for more peripheral lesions to be biopsied with greater accuracy.

INDICATIONS

- Lung transplant rejection surveillance and as clinically indicated
- Mass/nodule evaluation
- Mediastinal lymphadenopathy
- Inflammatory diseases
- Infections

EQUIPMENT

- Biopsy forceps
  - Size of forceps depends on the location of lesion and bronchoscope channel size
- Fluoroscopy, if using image guidance

PRE-PROCEDURAL PLANNING

1. Determining biopsy location
   - The most basic navigational technique requires pre-procedural planning; for example, reviewing prior imaging to identify potential target areas for TBB. This requires detailed knowledge of the bronchial branching pattern.

TECHNIQUE

1. Inspect the airway proximal to the planned biopsy location. Carefully clear secretions to the most distal aspect of the airway allowed by the bronchoscope.

2. Consider clearing the working channel by removing the bronchoscope and suctioning a small amount of normal saline through the suction port to prevent re-introduction of airway secretions when the biopsy forceps are advanced through the channel.

3. Confirm proper open/close function of the forceps prior to introducing the instrument into the working channel of the bronchoscope.

4. Align the tip of the bronchoscope in the center of a proximal airway, away from the bronchial mucosa. This allows a safe distance from the bronchial mucosa so the forceps can be visualized upon introduction. If introducing and advancing the biopsy forceps in a wedged position of the distal scope, you will be blinded from the forceps entering the lower airways with guidance primarily on fluoroscopy.

5. Introduce the biopsy forceps through the working channel slowly and smoothly, keeping careful watch on the bronchoscope tip on the video monitor. Fluoroscopy is used for biopsy guidance once the biopsy forceps has been deployed into the lower airways from the distal scope.

6. If the blind technique is being used from a wedged position, continue to advance the forceps into the subsegmental bronchus that leads to the desired biopsy location until resistance is encountered.

7. Once resistance is met, retract the forceps approximately 1–2 centimeters and attempt to open the biopsy forceps during inspiration. Dilation of airways during inspiration will aid in opening the forceps completely.

8. Advance the forceps until resistance is met. Then, have the assistant close the biopsy device.

9. Pull back on the forceps using quick, low-amplitude, moderate force to obtain a tissue sample.
   - If significant resistance is met while trying to obtain a biopsy, have the assistant open the forceps to release the sample. Then retract the forceps by about 1 centimeter, then close the forceps. Restart with step 6, attempting to take a smaller forceps bite.
   - If fluoroscopy is being utilized, make sure to stop active imaging at this step once the sample is obtained to avoid excessive ionizing radiation exposure.

10. Keeping the forceps closed, remove the sample from the working channel and deposit it in a sterile and biologically safe medium such as normal saline.

11. Repeat steps 3–10 with the same forceps to obtain multiple TBB samples. The amount and location of biopsies will be dependent upon the suspected, underlying pathology.

SAMPLE/SPECIMEN PROCESSING

- Excess saline should be removed, and samples should be transferred into a sterile container of 10% formalin if going for cytologic or immunohistochemical staining; however, processing protocols may differ based on the institution.
- Biopsies being sent for culture should instead be transferred to a sterile container of normal saline solution.

COMPLICATIONS (FREQUENCY, IF REPORTED)

- Hemorrhage/bleeding (1–4%)
- Pneumothorax (0.7–10%)
- Infection
- Oxyhemoglobin desaturations

PEARLS

- Lesions that are small, peripheral, or not situated near a bronchus bifurcation, known as the bronchus sign on computed tomography (CT), are typically more difficult to accurately biopsy. These should be avoided unless using more advanced techniques, such as CT-guided bronchoscopy or radial/linear endobronchial ultrasound (EBUS).
- We recommend the use of fluoroscopic guidance for transbronchial biopsies in order to reduce the risk of pneumothorax. This complication can be assessed following completion of the procedure.
- Post-procedure fluoroscopy may be useful to identify a pneumothorax, with chest imaging not being universally performed post-lung biopsy.
- Pulmonary hemorrhage can occur but can mostly be controlled by maintaining wedge pressure (reason to use the blind technique) and cold saline. If needed, oxymetazoline, epinephrine, and phenylephrine are agents we use to control bleeding. Management of a pulmonary hemorrhage is also discussed in Chapters 2 and 9.

FOREIGN BODY REMOVAL

Foreign body aspiration is a significant cause of morbidity and mortality in the pediatric population, and treatment will sometimes require medical teams to retrieve objects from the lower airways. Bronchoscopy provides a means for definitive diagnosis and management of foreign bodies. The urgency of bronchoscopic evaluation is dictated by patient clinical stability; rapid intervention in situations of precipitous decline can help to avoid serious sequelae of hypoxemia. Surgical experts skilled at managing airway complications should be notified prior to attempts at removing airway foreign bodies, in order to elicit timely assistance should difficulties be encountered during the procedure.

- Rigid bronchoscopy is commonly utilized for the retrieval of foreign bodies within the large central airways. Properties of the rigid endoscope allow for secure manipulation of foreign objects through a large working channel while simultaneously stabilizing the airway and providing ventilation. Further discussion of rigid bronchoscopy for the removal of foreign body is included in Chapter 9.
- Flexible endoscopes are useful for evaluation when small or fragmented objects are suspected of having migrated beyond the mainstem bronchi. Based on operator experience and the tools available, distally located foreign objects can be extracted from the airway or relocated to the mainstem bronchus *via* the flexible endoscope technique; the latter provides a route for ultimate removal of the foreign body by rigid instrumentation.
- There are a variety of devices available for use with both rigid and flexible endoscopes to retrieve airway foreign bodies, including suction devices, forceps, and endoscopic nets, snares, or baskets. If the size of the flexible bronchoscope working channel is large enough to accommodate a cryotherapy probe, this tool is also an option for removing some objects.
- BAL should be considered following removal of the object(s) when an infectious complication is suspected. Anti-microbials may be prescribed as part of the clinical management in patients considered to be at risk of infection.
- Additional considerations for post-procedural care may include maintenance of an artificial airway with continued mechanical ventilation and administration of systemic corticosteroids or bronchodilators. These interventions are employed when concerns about inflammation or bronchoconstriction arise. Many patients tolerate the procedure well and can be discharged home after recovery in the post-anesthesia care unit.

CONCLUSION

Rigid and flexible bronchoscopy are useful for evaluating the lower airways and lung parenchyma in pediatric patients with chronic respiratory symptoms. Flexible endoscopy allows for a more thorough inspection of structures distal to the mainstem bronchi and can facilitate procedures at the subsegmental airways. There are a variety of diagnostic and therapeutic interventions that can be performed through the flexible bronchoscope, and bronchoscopists can seek additional training in advanced procedures to enhance their interventional skillset. Complex procedures generally require intra-operative collaboration among surgeons and pulmonologists, so that pre-operative planning among multi-disciplinary airway teams remains essential to ensure that the goals of the evaluation are met.

TIPS FOR CLINICAL PRACTICE

1. Rigid and flexible bronchoscopes are utilized by surgical teams and pulmonologists to assess abnormal lower airway structure, obtain samples for pathology and microbiology analysis, and perform therapeutic interventions.
2. Flexible bronchoscopy is commonly employed for diagnostic investigation across the lower tracheo-bronchial tree, whereas rigid bronchoscopy is preferred for therapeutic interventions within the large central airways.

3. Airway secretions and tissues can be sampled through a variety of endoscopic procedures for the evaluation of chronic respiratory complaints and radiologic abnormalities.

4. Bronchoscopists comfortable with performing interventional techniques *via* the flexible endoscope can participate in specialized procedures at the lower airways, such as tumor debulking, foreign body removal, and airway stent or valve placement.

5. Potential consequences of lower airway endoscopy range from minor to serious and include fever, cough, transient hypoxemia, impaired ventilation, pneumothorax, bleeding, and bronchoconstriction.

6. Post-biopsy, visual evaluation for active bleeding can aid in limiting clinically significant hemorrhage.

7. Image guidance for transbronchial biopsies can detect and/or limit the complication of pneumothorax.

8. Multi-disciplinary pre-operative planning is essential to ensure that the goals of complex bronchoscopic evaluations are safely achieved.

9. Surgical checklists ensure that all required tools are available throughout the procedures.

REFERENCES

Alpert, BE et al. "Nonbronchoscopic approach to bronchoalveolar lavage in children with artificial airways." *Pediatric Pulmonology* vol. 13, no. 1 (1992): pp. 38–41.

Amitai, Y et al. "Serum lidocaine concentrations in children during bronchoscopy with topical anesthesia." *Chest* vol. 98, no. 6 (1990): pp. 1370–3.

Andersen, HA et al. "Transbronchoscopic lung biopsy in diffuse pulmonary disease." *Diseases of the Chest* vol. 48 (1965): pp. 187–92.

Balzar, S et al. "Transbronchial biopsy as a tool to evaluate small airways in asthma." *The European Respiratory Journal* vol. 20, no. 2 (2002): pp. 254–9.

Bossley, CJ et al. "Pediatric severe asthma is characterized by eosinophilia and remodeling without T(H)2 cytokines." *The Journal of Allergy and Clinical Immunology* vol. 129, no. 4 (2012): pp. 974–82. e13.

Bush, A, and P Pohunek. "Brush biopsy and mucosal biopsy." *American Journal of Respiratory and Critical Care Medicine* vol. 162, no. 2 Pt 2 (2000): S18–22.

Campbell, AM et al. "Functional characteristics of bronchial epithelium obtained by brushing from asthmatic and normal subjects." *The American Review of Respiratory Disease* vol. 147, no. 3 (1993): pp. 529–34.

de Blic, J et al. "Bronchoalveolar lavage in children. ERS Task Force on bronchoalveolar lavage in children. European Respiratory Society." *European Respiratory Journal* vol. 15, no. 1 (2000): pp. 217–31.

Eyres, RL et al. "Plasma lignocaine concentrations following topical laryngeal application." *Anaesthesia and Intensive Care* vol. 11, no. 1 (1983): pp. 23–6.

Faro, A et al. "Official American Thoracic Society technical standards: flexible airway endoscopy in children." *American Journal of Respiratory and Critical Care Medicine* vol. 191, no. 9 (2015): pp. 1066–80.

Goldfarb, S and J Piccione, editors. *Diagnostic and Interventional Bronchoscopy in Children.* 1st ed., Springer, 2021.

Londino, AV 3rd, and N Jagannathan. "Anesthesia in diagnostic and therapeutic pediatric bronchoscopy." *Otolaryngologic Clinics of North America* vol. 52, no. 6 (2019): pp. 1037–48.

McNamara, PS et al. "Comparison of techniques for obtaining lower airway epithelial cells from children." *The European Respiratory Journal* vol. 32, no. 3 (2008): pp. 763–8.

Miller, JI Jr. "Rigid bronchoscopy." *Chest Surgery Clinics of North America* vol. 6, no. 2 (1996): 161–7.

Paradis, TJ et al. "The role of bronchoscopy in the diagnosis of airway disease." *Journal of Thoracic Disease* vol. 8, no. 12 (2016): pp. 3826–37.

Pérez-Frías, J et al. "Normativa de broncoscopia pediátrica" [Pediatric bronchoscopy guidelines]. *Archivos de bronconeumologia* vol. 47, no. 7 (2011): pp. 350–60.

Pohunek, P et al. "Comparison of cell profiles in separately evaluated fractions of bronchoalveolar lavage (BAL) fluid in children." *Thorax* vol. 51, no. 6 (1996): pp. 615–8.

Rao, S et al. "Bronchial wash cytology: a study on morphology and morphometry." *Journal of Cytology* vol. 31, no. 2 (2014): pp. 63–7.

Ratjen, F, and J Bruch. "Adjustment of bronchoalveolar lavage volume to body weight in children." *Pediatric Pulmonology* vol. 21, no. 3 (1996): pp. 184–8.

Roden, AC et al. "Diagnosis of acute cellular rejection and antibody-mediated rejection on lung transplant biopsies: a perspective from members of the pulmonary pathology society." *Archives of Pathology & Laboratory Medicine* vol. 141, no. 3 (2017): pp. 437–44.

Tukey, M, and Lamb, C. "Bronchial washing, bronchoalveolar lavage, bronchial brush, and endobronchial biopsy." *Introduction to Bronchoscopy*, edited by A. Ernst and F. Herth, 2nd ed., Cambridge: Cambridge University Press, 2017, pp. 102–17.

Wood RE, Daines C. "Bronchscopy and bronchoalveolar lavage in pediatric patients." *Kending and Chernick's Disorders of the Respiratory Tract in Children*, edited by Wilmott RW, Bush A, Boat TF. 8th ed., Saunders, 2012, pp. 94–109.

Zavala, DC. "Pulmonary hemorrhage in fiberoptic transbronchial biopsy." *Chest* vol. 70, no. 5 (1976): pp. 584–8.

8

Advanced bronchoscopic procedures

KARTHIK BALAKRISHNAN AND R. PAUL BOESCH

DOI: 10.1201/9781003106234-8

INTRODUCTION

The earlier chapters of this textbook provide a discussion of the fundamentals and subtleties of upper and lower airway endoscopy. These chapters provide the reader with a foundation of knowledge and technique applicable to a wide variety of patients. In a minority of patients, more complex or unusual techniques may be helpful. These interventions require more complex instrumentation, devices, planning, and, in some cases, focused technical skill. This chapter will describe a selection of those techniques with brief discussions of patient selection, risks and pre-procedural counseling, necessary equipment beyond basic bronchoscopy, and clinical pearls drawn from the authors' experience collaborating in the care of many complex airway patients. Some of these techniques may be applicable to the "special situations" discussed in Chapter 9 as well. This chapter assumes a general understanding of flexible and rigid bronchoscopy, including fundamentals of instrumentation, setup, and technique; the chapter will focus on additional information that may be helpful to readers utilizing the advanced skills described here. Note that the authors strongly recommend photo and video documentation of all of these procedures.

ENDOBRONCHIAL ULTRASOUND WITH OR WITHOUT TRANSBRONCHIAL NEEDLE BIOPSY

Endobronchial ultrasound (EBUS) may be used for diagnosis as well as to provide imaging guidance for other procedures, such as transbronchial or transthoracic needle biopsy. EBUS developed from transesophageal ultrasound, when it was found that the non-echogenic airway lumen limited visualization of key mediastinal structures. EBUS was initially used mostly in lung cancer patients to visualize mediastinal lymph nodes and great vessels.[1] Since, then, applications have expanded to evaluation of airway wall infiltration, characterization of peribronchial and mediastinal masses and lesions, and imaging guidance for needle biopsy.

PREPARATION, POSITIONING, AND ANESTHESIA

EBUS is typically done *via* flexible bronchoscopy; it can be done *via* rigid bronchoscopy as well, though steering the flexible EBUS probe is more challenging in that setting. Positioning and anesthetic considerations are similar to other flexible bronchoscopic procedures. Consider working through an endotracheal tube if the patient is large enough to allow a tube that will pass the flexible bronchoscope. See the next section for further considerations of scope and tube size. All relevant imaging should be reviewed to allow the bronchoscopist to develop a mental map of where the lesion of concern lies relative to the airway. For paratracheal and parabronchial lymph node sampling, the appropriate stations for biopsy should be noted. Virtual or printed 3D models and virtual reality devices may help spatial understanding as well as patient counseling and team communication.[2] In all cases, the possibilities of airway obstruction, airway hemorrhage, airway rupture, and pneumothorax should be anticipated and discussed with the anesthesiologist ahead of time. A deeper plane of anesthesia may be warranted to decrease respiratory motion and cough reflex. These considerations apply to all procedures in this chapter and will not be recapitulated in each section.

EQUIPMENT

EBUS probes come in two types: radial and curvilinear. Each has strengths and weaknesses.[3] Briefly, radial EBUS uses a reusable flexible probe with rotating transducer that can pass through the working channel of a larger, flexible bronchoscope. The probe uses a saline-filled balloon to make contact with the airway wall. Currently available radial probes measure 1.4 mm in diameter and therefore can pass through a working channel as small as 1.7 mm. This allows the operator to use a relatively small bronchoscope (e.g., Olympus BF-MP190F bronchoscope, which has a 3-mm outer diameter at the tip, a 3.7-mm outer diameter of the insertion tube, and a 1.7-mm working channel). In turn, the bronchoscope size will determine whether the patient can be intubated for the procedure or whether the procedure must be done without intubation. The outer diameter of the insertion tube is greater than the tip and is what determines the size of endotracheal tube which can be used. This ability to use a small bronchoscope allows improved access to peripheral lesions, while radial EBUS also provides excellent visualization of the layers of the airway wall and beyond to a depth of about 4 cm. The major drawback of radial EBUS is that the probe occupies the working channel, preventing transbronchial needle biopsy or other instrumentation when the ultrasound is in position. However, the probe may be used to provide real-time guidance for transthoracic needle biopsy. The probe may also be passed *via* a sheath using fluoroscopic guidance, after which the sheath can be left *in situ* to guide any brush or needle biopsy instruments.

In contrast, the curvilinear probe is part of a fixed combination bronchoscope (EBUS-TBNA scope) that has a larger outer diameter of 6.9 mm (Olympus BF-UC180F). The tip of the bronchoscope incorporates a saline-filled balloon around the probe which must make contact with the airway. This device cannot be used in young or small patients, but it has the advantage of having a separate 2.2-mm working channel, allowing simultaneous instrumentation and ultrasound visualization. The device is shaped such that the biopsy needle to be passed through the channel will be aimed at the area shown by the ultrasound probe, with real-time visualization of the needle passage into the lesion.

TECHNIQUE

If radial EBUS is used, the bronchoscope should be guided as close to the lesion location as possible. The EBUS probe should then be passed through the working channel, relaxing the flexion at the tip of the scope and avoiding excessive insertion force that may damage the probe or scope. Under bronchoscopic visualization, the probe end is positioned in the airway lumen, and the probe balloon, if present, is inflated with saline to provide contact with the airway wall without any intervening air. If an endoluminal lesion is to be examined, the side of the probe is placed directly in contact with the lesion. If the bronchoscopist plans transbronchial or endobronchial biopsy, the probe can be placed through the working channel with a sheath. The sheath is left *in situ* once the probe is removed, to guide the biopsy instrument.

If curvilinear EBUS is used (**Figure 8.1**), the combination scope is passed into the airway lumen until the probe sensor can either be placed directly against the airway wall at the location of interest, or the balloon around the probe can be inflated at the location of interest. This is done until optimal ultrasound visualization is obtained. The scope is then allowed to relax to the neutral position. The biopsy needle device is passed

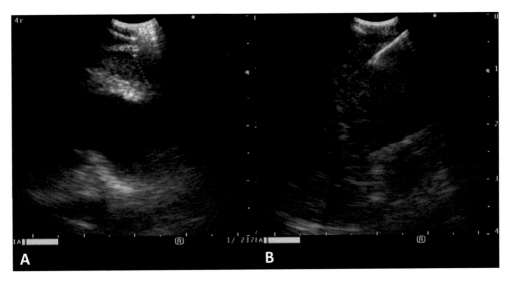

Figure 8.1 Curvilinear EBUS ultrasound measurement (A) and real-time needle aspiration (B) in a 16-year-old patient with suspected lymphoma.

into the working channel and locked into place, after which the integrated sheath is advanced until it is seen on bronchoscopic view. The sheath is locked into place and the scope again flexed to obtain optimal ultrasound view. The needle is then advanced through the sheath to sample the target lesion, the stylet is removed, and a syringe used to aspirate as the needle is moved within the lesion, in an even, jabbing motion. The syringe suction is released, the syringe is removed, and the needle is withdrawn. The scope is relaxed and the sampling setup removed. The sample is then acquired from the sampling device. Diagnostic yield is increased by taking multiple samples from each target station and further by utilizing a pathologist in the suite to prepare slides after each biopsy and assess for adequacy.

ENDOBRONCHIAL BIOPSY

Endobronchial biopsy, also known as transbronchial biopsy, is performed in a similar manner to the EBUS-guided biopsy technique described in the previous section. Both endoluminal lesions and extraluminal lesions adjacent to the airways may be accessed. The major difference is that conventional non-EBUS techniques rely on bronchoscopic visualization alone for guidance. Additional description of simple endobronchial biopsy is included in Chapter 7.

PREPARATION, POSITIONING, AND ANESTHESIA

This is the same as for EBUS-guided biopsy. In addition, the bronchoscopist should ensure that the chosen biopsy instrument will pass through the working channel of the flexible scope, or through the rigid bronchoscope if rigid airway access is part of the plan. If a rigid bronchoscope is to be used, the bronchoscopist should ensure that the rod telescope, any optical instruments, and rigid and flexible suction are appropriately selected to fit the rigid bronchoscope of choice.

EQUIPMENT

A standard flexible bronchoscope may be used to obtain endobronchial or transbronchial biopsies. Airway and endotracheal tube size will limit the size of scope that may be passed, in turn determining the size of the working channel.

As with EBUS-guided methods, a needle aspiration device may be passed through the working channel of the bronchoscope. In addition, a small biopsy forceps may be passed through the channel. Flexible biopsy forceps are available in a range of sizes that will fit through a working channel as small as 1.2 mm (e.g., Olympus FB-456D forceps). Like other uses of the working channel, simultaneous suction is generally not possible.

Flexible biopsy forceps are available with a variety of jaw shapes and lengths. One common variation is a "spike" between the jaws of the forceps. This allows the forceps to retain previously detached pieces of tissue by impaling them, permitting the operator to take two to three bites of tissue before removing the forceps. This may save time compared with non-spike forceps, which must be removed and the specimen retrieved after each bite in order to avoid loss of the specimen in the airway. Spike forceps are also advantageous in sampling lesions at an oblique angle as the tip of the forceps is anchored in the target and the jaws rotate to an angle more perpendicular to the lesion. These forceps require larger working channels. If the working channel size allows a choice between different forceps shapes, the bronchoscopist should consider the length of the jaws, which will determine how much the jaws can be opened in airways of different sizes, as well as the hinge action of the jaws. The latter will set how far out of the working channel the forceps must protrude to open (without damaging the bronchoscope), which, in turn, will determine how far from the bronchoscope the biopsy site must be kept and how easily the biopsy site is visualized while using the forceps.

Rigid bronchoscopy also allows biopsy. Steering flexible forceps through the larger lumen of the rigid bronchoscope and achieving any reasonable pressure on the airway carina or wall is challenging. Accordingly, rigid biopsy forceps, usually with cup-shaped tips, are often helpful. Optical cup forceps that incorporate a rod telescope may be particularly useful in providing both visualization and grasping ability; these will pass through size 3.5 and larger, rigid bronchoscopes or rigid tracheoscopes, keeping in mind that the size of rigid bronchoscopes does not explicitly communicate the inner or outer diameter of the scope. Rigid bronchoscopes also have the advantage of allowing the operator to pass a small suction catheter (e.g., Storz 5/6/7 Fr semi-rigid suction catheters) adjacent to the operating instrument within the lumen of the bronchoscope, allowing simultaneous suctioning and operating capability. Some catheters have a proximal Luer lock end, allowing either suction or irrigation as well as the application of other substances, such as fibrin glue.

TECHNIQUE

If the biopsy is to be performed through a flexible scope, the site is accessed as with standard flexible bronchoscopy. Endoluminal lesions should be clearly visualized. Topical vasoconstrictors (e.g., 1:20,000 or 1:50,000 epinephrine) may be applied preemptively to the planned biopsy site and allowed sufficient time (at least 2–5 minutes) to work before they are suctioned away.

If the lesion is extraluminal, the optimal site for biopsy *via* a flexible scope with forceps is at a carina, which allows straight-ahead visualization and puncture of the airway wall. The scope is positioned en face to the carina, after which the forceps are passed out of the working channel to a sufficient distance to allow them to enter the airway wall without soiling the scope tip and impairing visualization, yet close enough to provide stability to the forceps themselves; this placement may be challenging to achieve. The forceps are then either opened to grasp the carina to create a small opening in the cartilage wall, or (with larger and more rigid forceps) used to directly puncture the airway wall at the carina with the forceps closed. The forceps are then closed and passed through the opening just created in order to access the extrabronchial lesion.

If the lesion is adjacent to the airway wall but not at a carina, a needle can be passed through the flexible scope and used to puncture the airway wall at an angle, as with EBUS-guided biopsy. Alternatively, a rigid bronchoscope and rigid forceps may be used to puncture the airway wall at any location, carinal or otherwise.

When using forceps through the working channel of a flexible bronchoscope, it is often easiest to advance the forceps, open the jaws, pull the open forceps back close to the tip of the flexible scope, secure the position of the forceps in the scope at the biopsy valve, and then advance the whole scope and forceps together to the biopsy target site.

Once the biopsy sample has been acquired, any bleeding can either be allowed to stop spontaneously, controlled with topical medications, such as epinephrine as mentioned earlier, or controlled with a Bugbee flexible urologic cautery passed through a flexible or rigid bronchoscope. Any airway wall defect can either be allowed to heal spontaneously or it can be covered with a small amount of fibrin glue. If glue is used, it should never be applied through the working channel of a flexible scope, but through a separate catheter.

AIRWAY STENTING

The concept of stenting has been applied in surgery since the 1800s, and airway stenting was first used as early as 1872. Montgomery popularized the T-tube in the 1960s. Endoscopically deployed airway stents were initially adapted from endovascular devices but, over the past few decades, have evolved into their own range of technologies. Stents may be used in the airway lumen for a variety of purposes, including maintaining patency in stenotic, obstructed, compressed, or collapsible segments, supporting reconstructed areas of the airway, and covering defects in airway walls. Stents come in a variety of forms; this chapter will focus on hollow stents commonly used in the airway. Different stent types have not been directly compared in any study of reasonable quality, so the content in this section will be based on the authors' experience. Similarly, data are lacking on optimal indications for stenting and duration of stenting for the stents to be discussed here.

Stenting for static stenosis of the airway is most common in neoplastic narrowing in adult patients requiring palliative intervention, although we and others have used this technique for cicatricial narrowing of the airway in children as well. Stenting for dynamic intrinsic airway collapse (tracheomalacia or bronchomalacia) is less common. The largest study of this indication showed that, in 15 patients, 67% had improvement in symptoms.[4] New bioabsorbable stents may be helpful for this indication, as discussed later in this section. Stenting for extrinsic compression, for example from vascular structures, has been described in both adults and children.[5-7] The use of stents to cover tracheal or bronchial wall defects has been described in case reports[8,9] but not well studied.

PREPARATION, POSITIONING, AND ANESTHESIA

If a balloon is to be used, the anesthesiologist should be aware that a deeper plane of anesthesia is needed while the balloon is inflated and occluding the airway, in order to avoid barotrauma with coughing and negative pressure pulmonary edema with forceful inspiration.

EQUIPMENT

The bronchoscopist must first determine the type and size of stent suitable for the patient's specific need. In general, the first choice is between covered and non-covered stents. Non-covered stents are usually made of wire mesh or bioabsorbable materials. They have the advantage of allowing mucosal ingrowth through the openings in the stent wall, allowing continuity of mucociliary clearance. However, these openings also allow ingrowth of granulation, while mucosal coverage of the stent makes stent removal more challenging (but not impossible). Covered stents, in contrast, do not permit growth of mucosa or granulation within the stent and are much easier to remove. They may also be helpful in neoplastic narrowing of the airway because they allow less tumor ingrowth along the length of the stent. However, they impair mucociliary clearance over their length by covering the mucosa and may be prone to biofilm formation and mucus plugging. These stents may be made of wire mesh with a flexible covering, for example, the Atrium iCast, GORE VIABAHN VBX, and AERO stents, or they may be made of silastic/soft silicone, as with the Hood and Dumon stents. The authors prefer covered stents in most pediatric patients because the stent must typically be removed later, unlike the situation in many adult patients in whom palliative stents remain in place through to the end of life.

The bronchoscopist must also choose between self-expanding and balloon-deployed stents. The authors are not aware of any single stents that allow both methods of deployment. In general, self-expanding stents are easier to deploy, while balloon-expandable stents allow greater customization of diameter. Of note, some stents come pre-loaded on a balloon catheter, whereas others must be loaded onto a balloon by the operator.

The bronchoscopist must choose the appropriate stent diameter (inner and outer) and length. Some stents, particularly those with wire-mesh walls, will shorten as they expand in diameter. Typically, the packaging will indicate lengths at various diameters, and, for balloon-expandable stents, will sometimes also indicate the balloon inflation pressure needed to achieve these diameters. Length and outer diameter should be determined by imaging or careful direct measurement.

TECHNIQUE

Rigid bronchoscopy is generally the easiest way to deploy stents in airways proximal enough and which allow rigid access. The area to be stented is visualized using a rod telescope through the lumen of the bronchoscope. If a balloon-deployed stent or self-deploying catheter-delivered stent is to be used, the appropriate catheter is passed through the bronchoscope adjacent to the rod telescope and delivered into the airway. Ideally, the stent should be centered over the area of concern, though eccentric positioning may be needed to avoid impinging on the glottis or obstructing more distal airway branches.

If a self-expanding stent is used, the specific delivery system should be studied ahead of time to understand how and when the delivery catheter should be pulled back, and how the final stent location relates to the catheter tip position. Fluoroscopy may be helpful in placing these stents. The stent should be chosen such that its size allows secure placement without excessive pressure against the bronchial wall.

If a balloon is used to deploy the stent, the balloon should be inflated to achieve the desired stent diameter. Some stents may allow expansion beyond their nominal limit, but stent fracture is a risk. The balloon is then deflated and withdrawn to allow visualization of the stent (**Figure 8.2**). If parts of the stent need further expansion, this can be done. If the stent needs slight repositioning, this is best done with optical

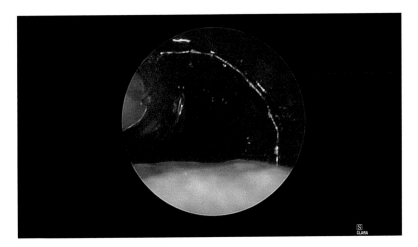

Figure 8.2 Balloon deflated and *in situ* after deployment of a wire-mesh stent in the trachea of a young adult with short-segment, congenital, tracheal stenosis following endoscopic laser division of a single complete tracheal ring.

forceps prior to final expansion. Once the full length of the stent has been expanded to the target diameter, the proximal end may be flared with a balloon 1 mm larger in diameter in order to engage the proximal tines into the mucosa and "lock" the stent in place, preventing cephalad movement with coughing (Figure 8.3). Overexpansion of the stent beyond this should be avoided, because increased pressure on the mucosa causes ischemia, which in turn promotes granulation tissue formation. The distal end of the stent usually should not be flared, because this makes removal more difficult.

The above stent types can also be placed *via* flexible bronchoscopy. In general, it is usually necessary to guide the balloon catheter through the larynx *via* direct laryngoscopy and then follow and guide the catheter with the bronchoscope. This procedure requires two operators, once for the scope and one for the balloon. Crimping or slightly curving the tip of the balloon catheter can help with steering, though excessive shape alteration may impair balloon inflation or deflation. An alternative is to use a flexible bronchoscope to pass a guidewire through the location to be stented. The stent-loaded balloon catheter can then be passed over the guidewire with the bronchoscope following behind to confirm appropriate placement. A large bronchoscope may allow passage of a balloon catheter through its working channel for subsequent additional dilation, although most balloons do not deflate tight to the catheter, so the entire bronchoscope must be withdrawn and the catheter cut to allow removal from the working channel.

If a silastic stent, such as a Hood or a Dumon stent, is used, it must be placed with rigid bronchoscopy. The stent is folded in on itself and grasped internally with alligator forceps to reduce its outer diameter (Figure 8.4), after which it is guided into position using the forceps and a telescope. When the alligator

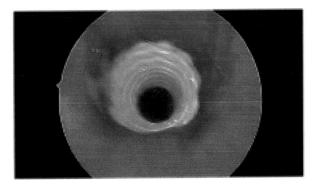

Figure 8.3 iCast stent deployed in the trachea of a 10-year-old patient with malignant destruction of the tracheal wall. Note the slightly flared, proximal end seated slightly into the mucosa without causing blanching.

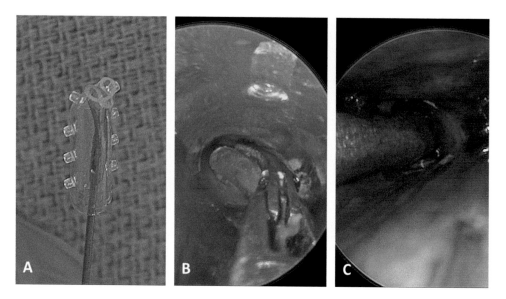

Figure 8.4 External (A) and internal (B) views of a silastic stent grasped from inside by rigid forceps. Placement of the silastic stent under direct visualization with rigid forceps and telescope (C). The stent was placed into the left mainstem bronchus of an infant with single-ventricle cardiac physiology and severe bronchial compression.

forceps are opened, the stent will expand and seat itself. Its proximal end can then be grasped to allow slight adjustment in position. Care must be taken when pushing it more distally, as airway injury may result. The alligator forceps can also be placed within the stent lumen and be opened to "pop out" any areas of residual stent infolding. It is initially more challenging to load the silastic stent in this way but there are distinct advantages over grasping the stent from the outside: the distal end of the stent is temporarily tapered to a narrower diameter, the trajectory of the stent is the same as the forceps themselves, and there is reduced risk of stent displacement when removing the forceps after deployment because the forceps are not between the stent and the airway wall.

MAINTENANCE

Stents are prone to shifting position, to obstruction from granulation or mucus, and to stent distortion or fracture (particularly with wire-mesh stents). Periodic bronchoscopy is necessary to assess and treat these issues. In some cases, periodic stent replacement is also helpful. With careful maintenance, stents in patients can be maintained for long periods. The first author (K.B.) has one pediatric patient with a nearly 5-cm tracheal wall defect (not currently reconstructable due to the patient's underlying disease) who has done well to date with a covered balloon-expandable stent for 18 months. Some clinicians use inhaled steroids or steroid–antibiotic combinations, inhaled bicarbonate, and other topical treatments to reduce granulation and biofilm formation (**Figure 8.5**). These measures have not been well studied and, while potentially beneficial, cannot replace periodic bronchoscopy.

ENDOBRONCHIAL VALVES

Endobronchial valves are one-way valves deployed within the airway lumen to isolate areas of the lung from airflow. These valves may be helpful in lung volume reduction for treatment of severe emphysema and have been applied in the treatment of bronchopleural fistulae.[8,9]

The valves are funnel- or umbrella-shaped devices, comprising a self-expanding wire skeleton and a membranous valve mechanism. The valves are delivered to the airway by a catheter, similar to some stents described earlier.

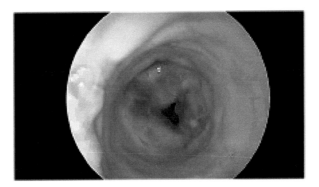

Figure 8.5 iCast stent after three months in the trachea without topical therapy in an 11-year-old patient with severe mid-tracheal tracheomalacia. Note the yellowish biofilm covering the stent as well as the distal granulation tissue, causing severe airway narrowing.

EQUIPMENT

Endobronchial valves are typically used in more distal airways as possible in order to avoid isolating entire lobes of the lung with a single valve; if a lobe is to be isolated, valves generally seat better in segmental airways that are valved individually (Figure 8.6). Accordingly, flexible bronchoscopy is usually the best tool to reach these airways. The deployment catheter requires at least a 2.6- or 2.8-mm working channel, depending on the valve system, which limits their use to larger, pediatric patients. Valve sizes are in the range 4–9 mm in diameter depending on the valve system used, with valve length increasing with increasing diameter.

TECHNIQUE

The flexible bronchoscope is positioned just proximal to the airway to be occluded. The valve kit comes with a calibrated sizing balloon that passed through the working channel and used to measure the diameter of the target bronchus. The balloon is deflated and removed, while the bronchoscope remains in position. A valve of

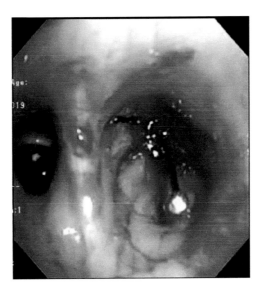

Figure 8.6 Endobronchial valves placed in three segmental bronchi of the right lower lobe in a 17-year-old patient with persistent bronchopleural fistula.

appropriate diameter is then loaded onto the delivery catheter and passed into position through the working channel. Note that, for most valve systems, the retention portion of the valve sits distal to the valve mechanism. The valve is delivered into the airway, ideally just distal to the take-off of the target bronchus. Placing the valve too close to the take-off may allow it to dislodge into the larger bronchus of the previous generation, while placing it too deep makes visualization and retrieval difficult.

ENDOBRONCHIAL BLOCKER

The endobronchial blocker (or "bronchial blocker") is essentially a balloon catheter designed to occlude rather than dilate an airway lumen. These devices are usually used intraoperatively for lung operations in patients for whom double-lumen endotracheal tubes are not a viable option, often due to size limitations.[10] Bronchial blockers may take more time to place and are more likely malpositioned than double-lumen endotracheal tubes, but carry less risk of sore throat, hoarseness, and mild airway injury.[11] Bronchial blockers may also be used to temporarily isolate lung regions for bronchopleural fistulae or airway hemorrhage, though, in the authors' experience, they do not generally maintain position and seal for long enough to provide useful temporization.

EQUIPMENT

Because the blocker is placed and left *in situ* with the catheter attached, it cannot be placed through the working channel of a flexible scope and may not be deliverable through smaller, rigid bronchoscopes, because in neither case can the scope be removed without removing the blocker. A flexible bronchoscope can be used to place the blocker, as can a laryngoscope and rod telescope. If a flexible scope is used, the blocker can be placed through an endotracheal tube or next to the tube. If passing through a tube, there must be sufficient inner diameter to accommodate the scope and the blocker side-by-side, which typically requires a small scope and a larger tube. If the patient has a tracheostomy, the blocker can pass through the tracheostomy tube, through the tracheostoma next to the tube, or through the mouth and larynx and then next to the tube. If the blocker is placed outside the endotracheal tube or tracheostomy, it may create an air leak around the tube cuff.

Bronchial blockers come in a variety of diameters and should be selected based on the size of the target airway.

TECHNIQUE

The bronchoscopist should determine whether the blocker can pass through the endotracheal tube or tracheostomy and still allow connection to a ventilator circuit. This is particularly problematic with tracheostomy tubes. Some blocker systems come with a Y-adaptor that allows connection to the circuit *via* one arm and an exit point that seals around the blocker catheter *via* the arm.

If passing through the tube, the blocker is first passed through the appropriate port on the adaptor, without connection to the tube itself. The bronchoscope is then passed through a bronchoscopic adaptor on the ventilation port of the blocker adaptor. A lasso loop on the blocker is then cinched tight around the distal end of the scope to secure it. The combination is then passed into the breathing tube and the adaptor connected to the tube and ventilator. The bronchoscope is used to guide the blocker into the target airway. The lasso loop is loosened and the scope pulled back slightly. The blocker is then inflated according to the product instructions to achieve the desired diameter, after which the inflation port is sealed according to the product instructions. The bronchoscope is used to confirm a good position. Fluoroscopy may be used to position the blocker as well. Some devices lock the blocker catheter in position within the Y-adaptor, which is attached to the endotracheal tube, to help prevent dislodgement.

If the blocker is in place for an extended period, it should be fully deflated and then reinflated at least twice a day to avoid gradual undetected deflation. Periodic bronchoscopic or radiographic position checks are also worthwhile.

CRYOTHERAPY

Cryotherapy involves the use of freezing and thawing to manipulate tissue. This may include variations such as cryoprobe, cryospray, and cryoadhesion.[12] Tissue freezing is created either by direct contact with a cold device or by topical application of liquid nitrogen. In general, tissues with a higher water content will be more affected.[12]

Cryotherapy may be used to ablate tissue, retrieve tissue and foreign bodies, and perform biopsies. Cryoadhesion involves directly contacting the target object, essentially freezing the tissue or foreign body to the end of the probe and allowing it to be pulled back partially or completely with the probe. Foreign bodies must have some water content in order to be removed with a cryoprobe. In the authors' experience, this method is also helpful for removal of large clots from the airway in the case of pulmonary or airway hemorrhage. Cryospray, in contrast, involves spraying the cooling substance or cryogen (usually a pressurized gas that causes rapid cooling as it exits the delivery device and expands) topically onto the target tissue, causing tissue damage and eventual necrosis and ablation.

EQUIPMENT

Cryotherapy requires a cryogen,. It also requires the actual delivery device, or cryoprobe, which may be rigid or flexible; flexible devices are generally more useful in the airways. Flexible cryoprobes are available in diameters as small as 1.7 mm, allowing use with both adult and larger, pediatric, flexible bronchoscopes.

TECHNIQUE

For cryoablation techniques, the bronchoscope is passed into the airway and positioned just proximal to the lesion of interest. The cryoprobe is passed through the working channel (or through the rigid bronchoscope) and advanced 5–10 mm past the tip of the scope to achieve contact with the lesion. The device is activated for several seconds and then deactivated. Further freeze–thaw cycles can be used to cause additional tissue damage and ablation. Visible freezing demarcates the area of damage, with the depth of injury measuring roughly 3 mm.[13] Because tissue necrosis and sloughing occurs in delayed fashion, repeat bronchoscopy may be helpful, and cryoablation may not be the optimal strategy for airway obstruction requiring prompt intervention.[12]

Cryoadhesion, in contrast, uses only the freezing portion of the cycle. Once the tissue has frozen to the tip of the probe, a brisk pull on the probe (in the case of biopsy or tissue removal) detaches a fragment of tissue that can be retrieved with the probe itself after it is thawed outside the patient. In the case of retrieval of an entire object (clots or foreign body), the probe is withdrawn more slowly to allow the entire object to follow the probe.

Cryospray, similar to cryoablation, ablates tissue through delayed necrosis. It has the advantage of creating a shallower depth of injury (1.5 mm[14]). It uniquely carries risks of inhalation of the cryogen deeper into the airway as well as barotrauma from rapid expansion of the gas.[12] Accordingly, the breathing circuit should be left open and the patient ideally kept apneic during application of the sprayed cryogen.[12] As with cryoablation, delayed bronchoscopy is needed to debride sloughing and necrotic tissue.

LASER

Lasers function by delivering light energy in the form of coherent, collimated, monochromatic, high-energy photons. They are available in many wavelengths, each with its own chromophore (tissue with increased energy absorption at a given wavelength, most commonly water or hemoglobin/blood). Most laser devices allow some control over the energy delivered, the duration and repetition of energy pulses, and the interval between pulses (or, in some cases, continuous delivery of energy). The energy delivered is measured in joules, with some lasers controlled in terms of rate of energy delivery (watts = joules/second). The effect of energy

Table 8.1 Common fiber-carried medical lasers applied in the airway

Laser	Wavelength (nm)	Chromophore
KTP	532	Hemoglobin
Nd:YAG	1064	Hemoglobin
CO_2	10600	Water

delivery can vary with the laser type, spot size, continuous *versus* pulse, and the energy delivered, and may include coagulation, incision/cutting, ablation, and cytotoxic effects.

Typically, bronchoscopists use fiber-delivered lasers *via* flexible fiber-optic cables. These can pass through either the working channel of a flexible scope or the lumen of a rigid scope; they can also be used with a variety of hollow, rigid handpieces that can be used in the proximal and mid (and sometimes distal) trachea with rod telescope visualization. Laser energy may be delivered to the tissue in either contact or non-contact fashion, depending on the laser.[15] Fiber-delivered lasers commonly used in the airway are listed in Table 8.1, along with their wavelength and chromophores that may be targeted during bronchoscopy. The bronchoscopist should select the appropriate laser based on the target tissue, such as the water and blood content of that tissue.

PREPARATION, POSITIONING, AND ANESTHESIA

All lasers carry a significant risk of airway fire, with potentially devastating or lethal consequences. Airway fires require three elements: a spark (laser energy), oxygen (delivered to the patient *via* the anesthesia circuit), and fuel (endotracheal tube, laser fiber sheathing, dessicated or charred tissue, etc.). All procedures involving lasers should include a pre-procedural discussion with the anesthesiologist and any procedural assistants or technicians covering the period in the procedure when the laser will be used, the need for both the inspired and the expired oxygen fraction to be less than 30% at that time,[16] assessment of fire risk using that institution's preferred scale, specific precautions to set up in case of fire, and designated roles in the event of a fire (e.g., anesthesiologist will cease oxygen and gas flow and disconnect circuit; bronchoscopist will pull endotracheal tube, technician will flood airway with saline, etc.). Care should be taken not to allow drapes or other materials to trap a cloud of oxygen around the patient that might ignite.

Immediately prior to each laser use, the inspired and expired fraction of oxygen should be confirmed as being less than 30% through direct discussion with the anesthesiologist, and emergency precautions and preparations should be reconfirmed. The patient should have wet gauze or laser-specific covers to protect the eyes, as well as coverage of the face and teeth to prevent burns from laser scatter. A "laser-safe" endotracheal tube may be used. These tubes typically have an external coating or wrapping that reduces flammability if struck with the laser, as well as a cuff inflated with blue-dyed saline to promptly indicate cuff rupture if struck by the laser. It is important to note that even "laser-safe" tubes may be ignited with sufficient energy delivery and surrounding oxygen.

EQUIPMENT

The appropriate laser generator and fiber should be available. Many lasers have more than one fiber diameter; the appropriate fiber should be chosen for the scope and application to be used. Some laser fibers require that the distal end of the fiber be "stripped" of its protective coating, using a specifically designed stripping device. Without this stripping, the outer coating may ignite, or tissue may adhere to the fiber tip in greater quantities and provide fuel for ignition. Appropriate handpieces, rigid bronchoscope, or flexible bronchoscopes should be selected; most laser fibers are quite thin and compatible with most working channel bronchoscopes, including the smallest pediatric scopes. All personnel in the procedure room should have wavelength-specific eye protection. If there is concern with respect to vaporization and aerosolization of tissue particles, a suction smoke evacuator device should be set up with its suction tube near the working field.

TECHNIQUE

The bronchoscope is passed into position and the appropriately stripped laser fiber threaded through the scope such that it protrudes slightly beyond the tip of the scope. An oxygen pause is conducted, appropriate protective draping confirmed for the patient, and protective equipment confirmed for all personnel in the room.

Non-contact lasers are used with the fiber tip sitting slightly above the lesion of interest. In some cases, holding the tip slightly farther from the tissue allows a wider delivery area for the laser energy, allowing more superficial action. Contact lasers, meanwhile, are placed lightly on the tissue. In some cases, as with the Nd:YAG laser for selected vascular lesions, the fiber may even be passed into the body of the lesion itself. The laser is usually activated by a pedal, with the amount and duration of energy delivered depending on the lesion and laser. In order to avoid unnecessary injury to adjacent structures, one should be mindful of respiratory motion, angle of approach, depth of penetration, and time of application. Deeper thermal injury cannot be seen and is more likely to occur with continuous rather than pulse mode.

Once the tissue has been adequately treated, charred tissue may have to be suctioned away or removed with biopsy forceps. With the CO_2 laser, in particular, but with all lasers to some degree, dry, charred tissue should be removed periodically. This tissue has little to no water or blood content and thus will simply heat up with further energy delivery, increasing the risk of ignition and also shielding the underlying tissue from being targeted.

CONCLUSION

Most advanced bronchoscopic techniques are useful in specific circumstances and may not be familiar to many bronchoscopists. However, they are conceptually straightforward and can be carried out safely and successfully with appropriate training, equipment, and preparation. Communication with anesthesiologists and other team members is essential, and in many cases a second operator will help the procedure proceed more smoothly.

TIPS FOR CLINICAL PRACTICE

- Many of the procedures described here can be performed through either rigid or flexible bronchoscopes. The choice depends on the specifics of the patient and the situation.
- Working with a calm, collegial, and expert anesthesiologist is extremely helpful. The concept of the "shared airway" comes into play nowhere more so than with these complex and sometimes high-risk endoluminal airway procedures. Advance discussion, communication, and planning are essential, as are careful discussion with the patient and informed consent.
- Virtual or physically printed 3D models are often helpful in procedural planning, communication with other clinical team members, and patient counseling and education.
- Photo and video documentation of procedures, as well as detailed note-taking immediately afterward, when the procedure is fresh in the bronchoscopist's mind, are helpful for training, education, personal review and improvement, and planning of procedures.

REFERENCES

1. Medford ARL. Endobronchial ultrasound: what is it and when should it be used? *Clin Med.* 2010 Oct; 10(5): 458–463.
2. Balakrishnan K, Cofer S, Matsumoto JM, Dearani JA, Boesch RP. Three-dimensional printed models in multidisciplinary planning of complex tracheal reconstruction. *Laryngoscope.* 2017 Apr; 127(4): 967–970.

3. Balamugesh T, Herth FL. Endobronchial ultrasound: a new innovation in bronchoscopy. *Lung India*. 2009 Jan-Mar; 26(1): 17–21.

4. de Trey LA, Dudley J, Ismail-Koch H, Durward A, Bellsham-Revell H, Blaney S, Hore I, Austin CB, Morrison GA. Treatment of severe tracheobronchomalacia: ten-year experience. *Int J Pediatr Otorhinolaryngol*. 2016 Apr; 83: 57–62.

5. Dodge-Khatami A, Backer CL, Holinger LD, Baden HP, Mavroudis C. Complete repair of Tetralogy of Fallot with absent pulmonary valve including the role of airway stenting. *J Card Surg*. 1999 Mar–Apr; 14(2): 82–91.

6. Arcieri L, Serio P, Nenna R, Di Maurizio M, Baggi R, Assanta N, Moschetti R, Noccioli B, Mirabile L, Murzi B. The role of posterior aortopexy in the treatment of left mainstem bronchus compression. *Interact Cardiovasc Thorac Surg*. 2016 Nov; 23(5): 699–704.

7. Barnes JH, Boesch RP, Balakrishnan K, Said SM, Van Dorn CS. Temporary bronchial stenting for airway compression in the interstage palliation of functional single ventricle. *Ann Pediatr Cardiol*. 2019 Sep-Dec; 12(3): 308–311.

8. Klooster K, Slebos DJ. Endobronchial valves for the treatment of advanced emphysema. *Chest*. 2021 May; 159(5): 1833–1842.

9. Gaspard D, Bartter T, Boujaoude Z, Raja H, Arya R, Meena N, Abouzgheib W. Endobronchial valves for bronchopleural fistula: pitfalls and principles. *Ther Adv Respir Dis*. 2017 Jan; 11(1): 3–8.

10. Moritz A, Irouschek A, Birkholz T, Prottengeier J, Sirbu H, Schmidt J. The EZ-blocker for one-lung ventilation in patients undergoing thoracic surgery: clinical applications and experience in 100 patients in a routine clinical setting. *J Cardiothorac Surg*. 2018 Jun 25; 13(1): 77.

11. Clayton-Smith A, Bennett K, Alston RP, Adams G, Brown G, Hawthorne T, Hu M, Sinclair A, Tan J. A comparison of the efficacy and adverse effects of double-lumen endobronchial tubes and bronchial blockers in thoracic surgery: a systematic review and meta-analysis of randomized controlled trials. *J Cardiothorac Vasc Anesth*. 2015 Aug; 29(4): 955–966.

12. DiBardino DM, Lanfranco AR, Haas AR. Bronchoscopic cryotherapy: clinical applications of the cryoprobe, cryospray, and cryoadhesion. *An Am Thorac Soc*. 2016 Aug; 13(8): 1405–1415.

13. Vergnon JM, Huber RM, Moghissi K. Place of cryotherapy, brachytherapy, and photodynamic therapy in therapeutic bronchoscopy of lung cancers. *Eur Respir J*. 2006 Jul; 28(1): 200–218.

14. Krimsky WS, Broussard JN, Sarkar SA, Harley DP. Bronchoscopic spray cryotherapy: assessment of safety and depth of airway injury. *J Thorac Cardiovasc Surg*. 2010 Mar;139(3):781–782

15. Verret DJ, Jategaonkar A, Helman S, Kadakia S, Bahrami A, Gordin E, Ducic Y. Holmium laser for endoscopic treatment of benign tracheal stenosis. *Int Arch Otorhinolaryngol*. 2018 Jul; 22(3): 203–207.

16. Remz M, Luria I, Gravenstein M, Rice SD, Morey TE, Gravenstein N, Rice MJ. Prevention of airway fires: do not overlook the expired oxygen concentration. *Anesth Analg*. 2013 Nov; 117(5): 1172–1176.

Bronchoscopy for specific situations

DOUGLAS SIDELL, CHRISTOPHER T. TOWE, AND MYMY C. BUU

INTRODUCTION

Both rigid and flexible bronchoscopy encompass a broad spectrum of procedures. These span the disciplines of pulmonary medicine, otolaryngology, critical care, and general surgery, among others. In the academic pediatric arena, there is often subtle overlap between procedures and specialties. Possibly of little surprise, few individuals perform all bronchoscopic procedures and instead tend to utilize bronchoscopy for purposes that lie within their own training and experience. Nevertheless, the past three decades have seen enhanced cross training between specialties and what is likely to be a significant improvement in patient care. This requires the dedicated bronchoscopist to understand the underlying principles of pulmonary bronchoscopy, laryngotracheal endoscopy, and other forms of interventional bronchoscopy alike. In addition, it requires a thorough understanding of the pathologic processes and training programs that define other disciplines outside of one's own specific training. Lastly, it requires an understanding of the equipment options available to perform bronchoscopy, the rationale for each endoscopic instrument's form and function, and the ability to appropriately apply these principles to the patient.

As suggested here, bronchoscopy is an incredible procedure and one that serves multiple purposes. It allows for a thorough diagnostic assessment of the patient's airways and has the ability to play an interventional and/or therapeutic role throughout the majority of the central airway and pulmonary tree. Hybrid approaches, using combined endoscopic techniques, either in tandem or in sequence, are also an important consideration. Airway endoscopy, however, is not without its limitations. Each instrument has its own catalog of benefits and shortcomings, all of which must be well known to the individual performing the procedure.

In this chapter, we aim to discuss a few key bronchoscopic procedures that are used in specific situations and hope to provide insight into the vast utility of airway endoscopy techniques and the importance of cross training and interdisciplinary collaboration. A large focus of this chapter will surround foreign body retrieval. Preparation, positioning, and anesthesia, as well as equipment and operating room (OR) setup details should follow the basic outline presented in Chapter 6. Additional details relevant to special situations are included in the sections below, though each list is by no means exhaustive.

FOREIGN BODY REMOVAL

PREPARATION

Although the decision to pursue bronchoscopy following a choking event is a key diagnostic consideration, it is beyond the scope of this chapter; however, when bronchoscopy is indicated, it is important to consider the following details prior to the procedure.

HISTORY

- **When did the foreign body aspiration or choking event occur?**
  - Events occurring within hours of bronchoscopy may be associated with fewer sequelae of chronic inflammation (**Video 9.1**). In contrast, in the setting of prolonged foreign body aspiration, the bronchoscopist must be prepared for the presence of sequelae, such as granulation tissue, bleeding, infection, and/or erosion of the airway(s) (**Videos 9.2 and 9.3**).
  - Over time, the foreign body itself may have changed in its consistency, size, appearance, and/or location since the initial aspiration event. Anticipating these possibilities is important, as it allows for the appropriate preparation of instruments and contingency plans prior to intervention.
  - The use of steroids such as dexamethasone or prednisolone may be indicated prior to bronchoscopy, particularly in the setting of prolonged foreign body aspiration events. This may reduce inflammation prior to attempts at retrieval.
  - Prolonged foreign body events may also raise the suspicion for violation of the airway lumen, which may not be apparent on initial physical examination and instead come to attention of the proceduralist upon removal.
- **What was the foreign body?**
  - Size, composition, number of foreign bodies, and the amount of time elapsed since aspiration are all important features. This information may directly influence the practitioner's selection of bronchoscope, optical grasping instruments, and approach to foreign body retrieval. Having the appropriate instrument available and ready prior to bronchoscopy is imperative. This reduces the need for instrument acquisition and setup during the procedure.
  - In the setting of food foreign bodies (e.g., nuts, legume seeds) it may be helpful to know if the foreign body was chewed prior to the choking event or aspirated whole. This information is not always available.
  - Certain foreign bodies require immediate removal based on the composition of the foreign body itself. Button batteries, when aspirated or ingested, are considered a surgical emergency, requiring immediate removal. The bronchoscopist should be prepared for significant tissue injury surrounding the foreign body itself, including eschar, tissue slough, and/or erosion of the airway (**Figure 9.1**).
  - Other events, such as aspiration of caustic substances, may produce tissue changes that are not readily apparent on initial bronchoscopy but continue to progress over time. The majority of these

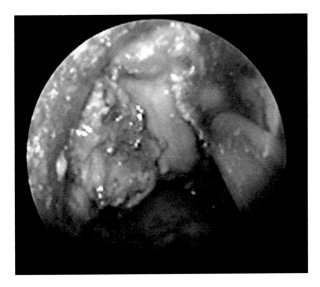

Figure 9.1 Tracheal lumen demonstrating eschar following button battery ingestion. Despite being swallowed, the battery created a tracheoesophageal fistula and was removed from the airway at the time of this photograph.

events are associated with laryngeal and pharyngeal burns but may necessitate an experienced airway specialist to establish and/or evaluate the airway (Videos 9.4 and 9.5).

- **Patient stability**
  - The decision surrounding the timing of bronchoscopic intervention is often dictated by patient stability and may be related in part to the timing of a foreign body aspiration event. Patients who ultimately present to the emergency room or outpatient clinical setting are, by definition, partial-obstruction events. Complete laryngeal or tracheal obstruction events, as may be seen in the setting of marbles, cellophane, or sausage aspiration, are either treated in the field or fatal prior to arrival at the hospital setting. Under some circumstances, a complete central airway obstruction may be partially dislodged and present thereafter as an incomplete obstruction event (Video 9.6). It is important to understand this history, as it may be predictive of recurrent obstruction or influence your bronchoscopic technique during removal.
  - In the stable patient and in the appropriate setting, a patient who has aspirated may be able to be observed safely for hours prior to removal. In contrast, a patient with inadequate ventilation, severe airway symptoms, or a compelling physical examination may require emergency intervention.
  - A general rule-of-thumb exists in that the patient's stability prior to presentation does not always preclude an urgent or emergency intervention. In other words, just because a patient has remained stable from the time of aspiration until the time of presentation does not always mean that continued observation or delay in treatment is appropriate. Ultimately, the decision to intervene should be made with the patient's safety at the forefront.
- **Patient age and weight**
  - The size of the patient is often influential when considering bronchoscopic technique and equipment choices prior to the procedure. Choosing the appropriate bronchoscope size (length and outer diameter) for the child's airway as well as the planned instrument(s) for retrieval depend on the available space both within the airway and within the bronchoscope.
  - Smaller airways may require a combination of techniques for foreign body removal and may preclude the use of larger optical grasping forceps. Likewise, both visualization and manipulation of the foreign body may be difficult in the smaller airway, particularly in the setting of bleeding, inflammation, or secretions.

- **Equipment decisions**
  - Both rigid and flexible bronchoscopes may be capable of removing small airway foreign bodies at a variety of locations throughout the airways. The decision is often made based on the aforementioned features surrounding the foreign body aspiration event, although having both rigid and flexible scopes available and ready during foreign body retrieval is prudent when possible.
  - The rigid bronchoscope allows for ventilation during evaluation and retrieval of the foreign body. It also provides the ability to stent the airway proximally and offers superior optics through the rigid telescope. Stenting of the airway can be seen in **Video 9.7**. The rigid bronchoscope is limited in its ability to reach smaller airways in the pulmonary tree (particularly in smaller patients) and relies on a single vector for visualization. Despite this limitation, the experienced bronchoscopist can often achieve exposure and foreign body removal from a variety of the segmental airways.
  - The smallest rigid bronchoscope through which an optical foreign body instrument will pass is a 3.5 bronchoscope. However, non-optical forceps can still be used effectively for foreign body removal in smaller pediatric or infant bronchoscopes. The ability to perform rigid bronchoscopy using the prismatic light source under direct visualization, rather than with the use of a rigid telescope, is an important skillset. This reduces the need for imaging monitors or cameras and can be performed with a single light source and ventilating circuit alone.
  - The flexible bronchoscope invariably has a smaller outer diameter than the rigid bronchoscope, thus allowing for the visualization of smaller or more distal foreign bodies. It allows for the wedged lavage of specific segments of the pulmonary tree (which may free some foreign bodies) and frequently has a working channel for a variety of flexible instruments (forceps, baskets, Fogarty catheters, etc.). The flexible bronchoscope may be used through the endotracheal tube (ETT) of an intubated patient *via* an adaptor, or, in the spontaneously ventilating patient, *via* a transnasal/ transglottic route. The patient is ideally intubated only after performing an evaluation of the central airway to reduce the risk of dislodging a central airway foreign body and pushing it distally. Shortcomings of the flexible bronchoscope include size limitations of the working channel, thus precluding the use of larger instruments, as well as a limited ability to ventilate the patient who is not intubated during the procedure. It is also important to remember that the flexibility of a pulmonary bronchoscope is reduced after insertion of an instrument through the working channel. Optics, although improving with distal chip technology, are inferior to the rigid endoscope.
- **Table layout**
  - *Avoid clutter.* Have your emergency airway equipment, including an appropriate range of bronchoscopes and ETTs, visible and organized on the side table.
  - *Assemble your equipment.* Do not plan to assemble your bronchoscope or optical forceps and telescopes "if you need them". Have everything ready. Have your flexible bronchoscope setup and ready before the patient arrives in the operating room.
  - *Check your telescopes and bronchoscopes.* Rigid and flexible scopes are fragile. Ensuring normal optics and visualization prior to starting the procedure is necessary.
  - *Include redundancy.* Expect equipment failure and have a contingency plan in place. Consider your light source, telescopes, bronchoscopes, optical instruments, and planned method of ventilating the patient.
  - *Prepare your optical and non-optical instruments.* As a rule of thumb, "If you think you may need it, have it open on the table". If you don't plan to use an instrument but there is even a small chance that such will be needed, have that item in the room and in a known location.
- **Personnel preparation**
  - Although emergency or urgent cases may not leave a large amount of time for pre-operative conversation, a brief huddle before foreign body removal is essential. If needed, this can be performed simultaneously during room setup and equipment preparation.

- Discuss the operative plan with the anesthesia team, nursing staff, and surgical technologist. Identify the roles of each person in the room and discuss anticipated procedural obstacles or patient-related concerns.
- Make sure each member of the team is familiar with the equipment that will be used for the case. Identify any shortcomings prior to the operation.
- Discuss airway management with the anesthesia team. At our institution, control of the airway is transferred to the otolaryngologist at the beginning of the procedure and the table is turned 90 degrees away from the anesthesia cart. Airway management is a shared endeavor and open communication is key.

- **Performing the procedure**
  - Ideally the patient is maintained spontaneously ventilating throughout the procedure. Mask ventilation assistance can be provided with the understanding that positive airway pressure may influence the location or position of the foreign body.
  - When the patient is adequately sedated and spontaneously ventilating, a "first-pass" rigid endoscopy can be performed. This is frequently done with a zero-degree rigid endoscope, passed transorally and trans-glottically with a conventional laryngoscope in place. This allows for evaluation of the central airway and identification of the foreign body.
  - Foreign bodies that have minimal surrounding inflammation and are amenable to removal with an optical forceps can then be removed either directly (using the optical forceps alone), or by first inserting a rigid ventilating bronchoscope and then removing the foreign body through the bronchoscope.
  - Prior to removal, the size and composition of the foreign body must be considered after it has been inspected. Large foreign bodies, particularly nuts and toy parts, may have passed through the cricoid under significant negative intrathoracic pressure. For this reason, they may be more difficult to remove. With an optical grasper surrounding the foreign body, it may be difficult to fit through the narrow and rigid cricoid lumen with the added outer diameter associated with the grasper (**Video 9.8**). Planning for this possibility prior to bringing the foreign body to the level of the larynx is critical. If the foreign body is brought to the cricoid and is unable to pass, it should be immediately replaced in a unilateral bronchus or distal central airway (if space is available to ventilate around it) while another plan is decided upon. Softer, malleable foreign bodies may be able to be broken into smaller pieces and removed individually.
  - Rarely, larger solid foreign bodies (often toys or toy parts) require removal *via* a tracheostomy. This requires a two-team approach, with the tracheostomy being created by one surgeon while the other manages the airway with a rigid bronchoscope, if needed. The foreign body can then be grasped endoscopically, brought to the central airway, and immediately removed through the surgical stoma. Under even more rare circumstances, larger or centrally obstructive foreign bodies such as marbles, may require distalizing of the foreign body or removal *via* thoracotomy or thoracoscopy. Lastly, a thoracic approach may be needed for patients with foreign bodies wedged in distal segmental airways that are not able to be effectively removed with a flexible bronchoscope, or that have migrated out of the airway lumen.
  - Foreign bodies that are located centrally (in the trachea or larynx) and are partially obstructive may be removed using a multitude of techniques. If the object is located at the level of the larynx and the patient is stable, the foreign body may be able to be grasped and removed under direct visualization. Alternatively, suspension laryngoscopy can be performed. This is an uncommon requirement, but, when tolerable, suspension allows for two-hand manipulation of the airway and foreign body, and removal with optical or non-optical forceps. Occasionally, passing a small right-angle probe beyond the foreign body, and pulling the probe out of the airway with the foreign body itself can be performed. Other techniques, such as using a Fogarty catheter or airway balloon, have been used to dislodge a laryngeal foreign body. At any time, if the patient becomes unstable, breaking

up the foreign body (if possible) and/or distalizing it to a larger airway or unilateral bronchus may be indicated. At the level of the larynx, the cricoid is the narrowest segment of the airway. If the foreign body is too large to pass beyond the cricoid, attempts to push distally may wedge it in a position the precludes removal, and may lead to complete airway obstruction.

- When using a flexible bronchoscope to remove a foreign body, small cup forceps, urologic retrieval baskets, cryotherapy probes, and/or Fogarty catheters may be employed to either assist in removal or to achieve complete removal of the foreign body. All have proven benefit under select circumstances, but none are universally effective.

- Flexible bronchoscopy is often helpful in bypassing granulation tissue, and also allows for gentle on-demand intermittent insufflation (by entraining low-flow oxygen through the suction port), if needed. It can be used in sequence with rigid endoscopy, or in tandem (through the lumen of the ventilating bronchoscope) under select circumstances.

- **Following foreign body removal**
  - After all foreign bodies have been removed, a thorough airway evaluation must be performed. This allows for documentation of airway inflammation or other sequelae of the foreign body aspiration event (or sequelae from removal). This is often done with a flexible bronchoscope, which can also rule out any other smaller, more distal foreign bodies. It also allows for the direct instillation of topical medications or fluids such as epinephrine, oxymetazoline, or saline if needed.
  - Occasionally, the entire foreign body and/or all of the foreign bodies aspirated may not be able to be removed. This may require interval stabilization, treatment with anti-inflammatory measures, and return to the operating room at a future point in time. Anti-inflammatory measures may include nebulized steroid/antibiotic solutions (e.g., ciprofloxacin/dexamethasone), systemic steroids, or racemic epinephrine, to name only a few.
  - The decision to extubate at the conclusion of the procedure depends on patient stability and the appearance of the airway following removal of the foreign body. The majority of patients do well after foreign body removal when extubated and spontaneously ventilating; it is uncommon for a patient to require post-operative intubation. However, physiologic or anatomic characteristics such as post-obstructive pulmonary edema (POPE), severe airway edema, or bleeding, may require a period of post-operative intubation and mechanical ventilation.

Video 9.1 Rigid endoscopy (Hopkins rod) demonstrating a peanut foreign body in the right mainstem bronchus. The foreign body had been present for 90 minutes at the time of the video.

Video 9.2 Removal of granulation tissue surrounding a peanut foreign body that had been present for 14 days at the time of the video.

Video 9.3 Following removal of the granulation tissue (Video 9.2); a peanut foreign body is visualized in the left mainstem bronchus surrounded by inflammation.

Video 9.4 Laryngoscopy demonstrating mucosal injury 24 hours after ingestion of lye.

Video 9.5 Laryngoscopy demonstrating severe scarring and mucosal changes surrounding the larynx and hypopharynx 6 weeks after ingestion of lye. This is the same patient as seen in Video 9.4.

Video 9.6 Severe inspiratory retractions and laryngeal obstruction visible on laryngoscopy and rigid bronchoscopy.

Video 9.7 Rigid ventilating bronchoscopy. This patient does not have an airway foreign body present; however, the video demonstrates the ability of the rigid bronchoscope to stent the airway proximally and provide simultaneous ventilation.

Video 9.8 Removal of a peanut foreign body using optical forceps. Note that the foreign body meets resistance with the optical forceps in place at the level of the cricoid cartilage.

LARGE-VOLUME/MASSIVE PULMONARY HEMORRHAGE

Many disease processes may lead to pulmonary hemorrhage. These include a myriad of diseases leading to diffuse alveolar hemorrhage syndrome (DAH), including infectious, malignant, and inflammatory etiologies. This section will focus only on bronchoscopic intervention associated with large-volume pulmonary hemorrhage or central airway bleeding events.

INITIAL MANAGEMENT

- **Protection of the airway and volume resuscitation**
  - If the source of bleeding is known/suspected, and the source is unilateral, place the patient in a lateral decubitus position with the bleeding side down.
  - For large-volume events, fluid/volume resuscitation efforts should ensue in parallel with bronchoscopy.
- **Single-lung intubation**
  - Single-lung intubation can be performed with an ETT or rigid bronchoscope. If an ETT is placed or already present, this may be accomplished using a flexible bronchoscope through the ETT.
  - It is recommended to use a bronchoscope with the largest working channel to allow for suction of active bleeding to ensure adequate visualization.
  - If the right lung is the source of bleeding, intubation of the left lung is often acceptable and can be achieved with a standard or microcuff ETT.
  - If the lumen of the bronchus is narrow, a smaller than age-appropriate tube may be required. If the smaller ETT is too short, a longer tube can be created by suturing two ETTs together over a cut ETT adaptor (**Figure 9.2**).
  - If the left lung is the source of bleeding, intubating the right lung may not provide adequate ventilation, as the right upper lobe bronchus may be bypassed or obstructed. Instead, placement of a bronchial blocker in the left mainstem bronchus followed by central/tracheal intubation may be required (**Video 9.9**). This can be done alongside the ETT or, in larger airways, through an ETT

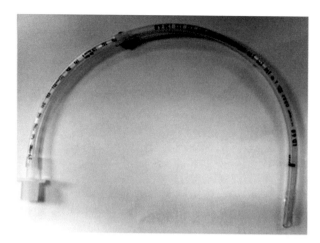

Figure 9.2 A custom extended-length microcuff endotracheal tube used for left mainstem intubation. Note the cut adaptor adjoining the two tubes, sutured in place using prolene sutures. *In situ*, the adaptor remains supraglottic to reduce the risk of granulation tissue formation or airway irritation. (Adapted from design by Michael Rutter, MD, SF. Cincinnati Children's Medical Center.)

alongside the bronchoscope. If placed alongside the bronchoscope within the ETT, a smaller bronchoscope is often required.

- If a bronchial blocker is not available, a Fogarty catheter may be adequate to provide temporary bronchial blockade.

- **Bilateral massive pulmonary hemorrhage**
  - If the source of bleeding is bilateral, the volume of bleeding and ventilatory status must be assessed. If a source cannot be identified and inadequate ventilation ensues, extra-corporeal membrane oxygenation (ECMO) or an alternative means of oxygenation must be considered early.

- **Rigid *versus* flexible bronchoscopy**
  - Flexible bronchoscopy allows for selective intubation and bronchial blockade as described. It allows for the identification and potential management of slower-flow distal segmental bleeding sources.
  - Flexible bronchoscopy is limited by the diameter of the suction channel and may not provide adequate visualization during large-volume brisk bleeds (**Video 9.10**).
  - Rigid bronchoscopy is often safer and is more effective at clearing blood and clot from the airways. It allows for simultaneous ventilation and has superior optics. The telescope can be removed and cleaned without removing the ventilating bronchoscope. A large suction catheter can be passed via the ventilating bronchoscope (**Figure 9.3**), and a flexible bronchoscope can be passed *via* the lumen of the rigid ventilating bronchoscope (hybrid approach), if needed.
  - Rigid bronchoscopy can bypass or tamponade bleeding sources in the setting of large-volume bleeds such as tracheo-vascular fistulae. Rigid bronchoscopy allows for bronchial blocker placement while maintaining control of the airway and concurrently suctioning active bleeding during the procedure.

- **When to stop**
  - When the patient is stabilized and the source of the bleeding is identified and quelled (not necessarily stopped completely), it is appropriate to re-assess the patient.
  - Dissolving a clot may be mistaken for active bleeding, and suctioning/clearing all the clot at that time is not always appropriate as this may stimulate additional brisk bleeding following clot removal.

- **Next steps**
  - Large vascular bleeds (e.g., tracheo-innominate fistulae) may require interventional radiology or an open-surgical approach to treat. These bleeds are often fatal but may be tamponaded by means of a precisely placed ETT, rigid bronchoscope, or (in tracheotomized patients) by maintaining pressure

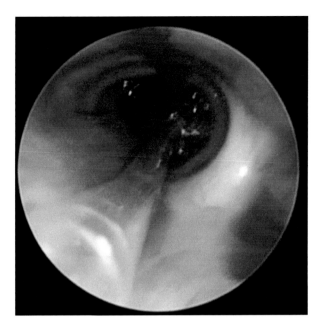

Figure 9.3 Rigid ventilating bronchoscopy used during pulmonary hemorrhage. A large suction catheter maintains a patent airway and promotes visualization during the procedure. The patient is ventilated simultaneously through the bronchoscope.

on the bleeding source through the stoma with an ETT or (rarely) small finger. The airway is maintained actively throughout transport and until the source of bleeding is repaired or controlled endovascularly (**Video 9.11**; **Figures 9.4** and **9.5**).

- Smaller, more distal bleeding sources may require endoluminal adjuncts to stop an active bleed.

- **Endoluminal adjuncts**
   - Topical epinephrine or other vasoconstrictors (e.g., oxymetazoline) may be considered for isolated bleeding events, although this is frequently done after bleeding has largely been controlled. This does not treat large-volume sources and has the potential to alter cardiac function.
   - Electrocautery can be performed focally using a flexible cautery probe (e.g., Bugbee cautery) advanced through the working channel of a rigid or flexible endoscope. Combustion/fire risk must be taken into account (**Video 9.12**).
   - Laser therapy has been effective in the setting of bleeding endoluminal sources such as neoplastic masses. The ND-YAG has the ability to stop or reduce bleeding but also has the ability to cause injury to surrounding structures.
   - Argon plasma coagulation, which utilizes an electrical current through a probe and is conducted by blood, can slow or stop smaller bleeding sources with arguably reduced potential for concomitant injury to deeper tissues.
   - Cold saline lavage has been performed with some success, often through a rigid bronchoscope and performed with 3–4° C saline. The rigid bronchoscope can continue to clear clots and control bleeding immediately prior to lavage. The volume of saline instilled, frequently based on patient weight and lung volume, must be considered.
   - Antidiuretic hormone (ADH) and derivatives can be used to control small-volume sources. This is thought to be as effective as epinephrine but with a lower potential for cardiac sequelae. Depending on the institution and/or location of the patient at the time of the bleed, ADH derivatives may not be as readily available as topical epinephrine, and this may limit their utility in emergency situations.
   - Cryotherapy has the ability to stop bleeding and may serve as a useful adjunct to remove clots. This is particularly useful for cessation of bleeding if an endoluminal neoplasm is identified and if

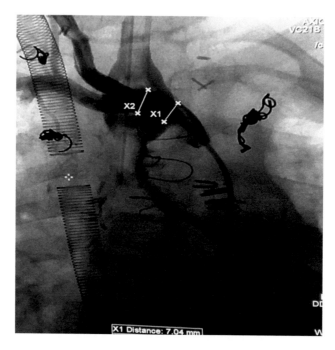

Figure 9.4 Endovascular management of a tracheo-innominate fistula. Note the contrast bronchogram created due to bleeding into the airway prior to the time of stent placement and image acquisition.

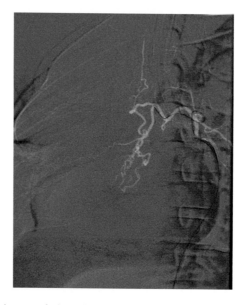

Figure 9.5 Endovascular evaluation of a bronchopulmonary malformation presenting with pulmonary hemorrhage. Note the collateral branch to the vertebral artery, precluding coiling.

bleeding is not profuse. Cryotherapy leads to vasocontriction and capillary thrombus formation, reducing or stopping active bleeding. It also has the ability, following control of bleeding by other methods, to remove clots. The cryoprobe can adhere to clots that are difficult to extract and assist in removal from the lumen during subsequent pulmonary clearance procedures.

– Other adjuncts, such as fibrinogen/thrombin mixtures and tranexamic acid, have been used to treat or prevent bleeding from patients with mucosal bleeding events, particularly if a bleeding disorder or anticoagulated state exists. Fibrinogen may be applied *via* a flexible or rigid bronchoscope, although flexible bronchoscopy is often preferred. This can be instilled after a cold saline lavage at the site of previous bleeding, and after most of the bleeding has stopped. Recombinant activated factor VII can be directly instilled for diffuse pulmonary hemorrhage.[1]

Video 9.9 Bronchial blocker placement in a unilateral mainstem bronchus.

Video 9.10 Active bleeding during flexible bronchoscopy. Note the inability of the bronchoscope's suction channel to clear the airway adequately in this patient.

Video 9.11 Laryngoscopy and rigid endoscopy demonstrating an active tracheo-innominate fistula in a 4-year-old child. The bleeding was controlled with a 14F suction catheter, and the endotracheal tube was advanced to reduce the vascular flow by placing the cuff of the tube at the location of the fistula. The fistula was endovascularly treated.

Video 9.12 Rigid bronchoscopy with electrocautery of the airway lumen.

THE AERODIGESTIVE PATIENT AND COMBINED ENDOSCOPY

Patients with complex laryngeal, tracheal, and pulmonary diseases frequently require the experience and expertise of both the pulmonologist and otolaryngologist, among others. A combined diagnostic aerodigestive evaluation frequently includes a "double endoscopy" (pulmonary flexible bronchoscopy and rigid laryngoscopy and bronchoscopy) or "triple endoscopy" (pulmonary flexible bronchoscopy, rigid laryngoscopy and bronchoscopy, and esophagogastroduodenoscopy [EGD]). The order of such procedures is an important consideration when attempting to identify aerodigestive pathology. These combined endoscopic procedures demonstrate the unique characteristics of each scope and/or technique. This description is not exhaustive.

- **Rationale for double and triple endoscopy**
  - These procedures allow for the pulmonologist, otolaryngologist, and gastroenterologist to work side-by-side in the operative arena to investigate aerodigestive pathology. The experience brought from each discipline and through each technique provides a synergistic diagnostic experience. This has been shown to: (1) enhance communication between providers; (2) improve one's understanding of the relationship between disease processes throughout the aerodigestive tract; and (3) reduce operative time and exposure to general anesthesia.
  - These procedures require appropriate communication with the anesthesia provider to achieve optimal sedation and patient safety throughout.
- **Order of procedures**
  - Double and triple endoscopy can be performed in sequence, or simultaneously.
  - When in sequence (the most common situation), the evaluation begins with flexible bronchoscopy *via* a transnasal, transglottic route. This requires the lowest amount of sedation and allows for the dynamics of the airway to be assessed.
    - The dynamic airway assessment begins with a "sleep state endoscopy", visualizing the dynamic appearance of the nasal airway, nasopharynx, hypopharynx, and larynx in the absence of a laryngoscope blade or excessive sedation (Video 9.13).

- Beyond the level of the larynx, in the minimally sedated and spontaneously patient, the dynamic motion of the trachea, bronchi, and lower airways can be assessed throughout the respiratory cycle, and during stimulated cough (**Video 9.14**).
  - Bronchoalveolar lavage, if indicated, can also be performed.
- Laryngoscopy and rigid bronchoscopy are performed following pulmonary bronchoscopy. This requires a deeper level of sedation due to the stimulus associated with laryngoscope placement.
- Rigid endoscopy allows for manual palpation of the laryngeal structures and accurate sizing of the subglottis using a variety of methods. This also allows for interventions, such as balloon dilation of stenotic segments of the larynx and trachea, cautery of recurrent tracheoesophageal fistulae, and endoluminal stent placement, among others.
- Larger-diameter suction catheters can enhance airway clearance using the rigid bronchoscopic technique.
- When using a ventilating bronchoscope rather than a rigid telescope alone, ventilation can also be achieved, if needed. In the pediatric aerodigestive arena, patients are commonly maintained spontaneously ventilating. A ventilating bronchoscope is rarely needed for diagnostic purposes.
- At the conclusion of the procedure, the patient can be intubated with an age-appropriate ETT prior to EGD. It is important to perform a thorough evaluation of the airway in a patient with potential pathology prior to intubation.
- **Simultaneous endoscopy**
  - Simultaneous bronchoscopy and esophagoscopy can be performed in the setting of communicating pathology, such as tracheoesophageal fistula (TEF) or laryngotracheal cleft (**Figure 9.6**). Insufflation of the esophagus, while observing the lumen at the site of a previously repaired TEF, may yield persistent communication that is otherwise elusive.

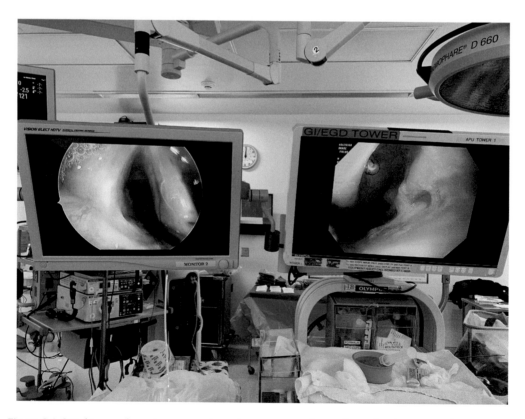

Figure 9.6 Simultaneous bronchoscopy and esophagoscopy can be performed in the setting of communicating pathology.

- Other forms of hybrid endoscopy include flexible bronchoscopy through a ventilating broncho-scope. This can be performed in the setting of patients requiring intermittent ventilation and the use of rigid instrumentation, but who also may require interval evaluation or clearance of the distal pulmonary tree.

Video 9.13 Sleep endoscopy using a pulmonary bronchoscope, demonstrating mild glossoptosis and bilateral pharyngeal collapse.

Video 9.14 Severe tracheomalacia visualized with a flexible bronchoscope in a spontaneously ventilating child.

TRAUMATIC AERODIGESTIVE INJURIES

Traumatic aerodigestive injuries encompass a broad spectrum of pathology, including caustic ingestion, tracheal laceration, tracheobronchial disruption or stenosis, and iatrogenic or traumatic tracheoesophageal fistula formation. This section will focus only on traumatic injuries that involve violation of the endoluminal airway.

- **Initial management**
  - In a fashion similar to pulmonary hemorrhage, initial management includes stabilizing the patient, identifying the location of injury, and subsequent treatment of the injury. In the setting of pneumothorax, with or without tamponade, chest tube placement may be required emergently.
  - If a patient is not intubated and appears stable, maintaining spontaneous negative pressure ventilation is often ideal. Unfortunately, tracheal or bronchial laceration, stenosis, and/or disruption are often the result of extensive injury or polytrauma, and mechanical ventilation is frequently required. This may result in extensive subcutaneous emphysema, supporting the diagnosis of an airway (or esophageal) injury.
  - In a patient with a high central airway or laryngeal injury, intubation or translaryngeal bronchoscopy may not be possible until tracheostomy is performed. This is particularly true in any patient with a suspected laryngotracheal separation or complex laryngeal fracture.
  - If a patient is stable for imaging, this may provide useful information pertaining to the location or extent of injury. Nevertheless, the patient must be thoroughly evaluated for stability prior to making this decision, as an airway emergency in the radiology suite may limit your ability to intervene adequately. If advanced imaging studies are obtained (e.g., computed tomography), an experienced airway provider and/or surgeon should accompany the patient during acquisition.
- **Airway evaluation**
  - Airway evaluation should be performed in the safest possible environment. This is frequently the operating room, although it may include an intensive care unit setting under select circumstances. The severity of injury and stability of the patient may dictate the location of intervention.
  - *The non-intubated patient*
    - If unstable, an emergent airway evaluation must be considered. Direct laryngoscopy and rigid bronchoscopy (using a rigid endoscope or ventilating bronchoscope) can be performed rapidly.
    - If severe laryngeal trauma is identified or laryngotracheal separation is suspected, emergent tracheostomy should likely be performed prior to completing the airway evaluation.

- If a tracheal or bronchial defect is identified, an ETT can be placed over a rigid telescope and passed beyond the defect or into a mainstem bronchus. If the injury is located at the carina, left mainstem insertion and single-lung ventilation may be required.
- Esophagoscopy should be performed once stabilized to ensure that esophageal injury is not present. This is particularly true in complex injuries, penetrating injuries, and under circumstances where the airway evaluation does not account for the free air identified on imaging or physical examination.
  - Left mainstem injuries, injuries with esophageal involvement, complete bronchial separation, and/or any injury which is not able to be bypassed may require emergent surgical repair. If the patient is unstable, air extravasation cannot be avoided, and/or it is unable to adequately ventilate, an alternative means of oxygenation (e.g., ECMO) must be considered.
  - *The intubated patient*
    - Flexible bronchoscopy through an existing tube is arguably the least-invasive and highest-yield approach in the intubated patient. The ETT may need to be withdrawn partially to identify the location of injury (Video 9.15).
    - It is important to avoid insufflation or high-pressure ventilation proximal to the site of injury, as this may promote air extravasation and limit the ability to ventilate the patient.
    - Avoid over-suctioning the area of injury or probing with the flexible bronchoscopy. A partial-thickness injury may be propagated.
    - Be cognizant of the level of sedation/anesthesia during the procedure. Topical anesthetic should be used, when possible, as triggering cough may exacerbate injury in the setting of luminal laceration or airway disruption/separation.
    - If the ETT has been withdrawn, it is important to place the ETT beyond the level of injury following evaluation. Avoid false passaging the ETT upon re-insertion. Having a rigid endoscope or bronchoscope at the ready in the event that the ETT cannot be easily passed beyond the luminal defect is prudent.
    - Once the location and extent of the injury are identified under direct visualization, rigid endoscopy may be warranted for improved visualization and/or intervention.
- **Intervention**
  - In the absence of the acute need for surgical intervention, many tracheal and bronchial lacerations will heal spontaneously over a short period of time (1–2 weeks).
  - The ability to bypass the injury and avoid air extravasation, and to maintain adequate ventilation and/or provide an alternative means of oxygenation often define non-operative injuries.
  - If the lesion is at the carina or mainstem bronchus and unilateral lung intubation is required, interval evaluation of the bypassed lung and clearance of the tracheobronchial tree at routine intervals during the healing process is prudent.
  - To bypass an injury, a microcuffed ETT or custom ETT may be required.
  - Stent placement to breach an area of injury may be considered, although this infrequently prevents air extravasation and may propagate injury. This should be performed with caution and the stent should be checked frequently, if placed.
  - Bronchial injuries which result in complete stenosis during healing (or as the sequelae of prior unidentified injury) likely require excision and bronchoplasty.
    - Balloon dilation using a rigid or flexible endoscope may be useful under select circumstances to avoid complete stenosis.
    - Endoluminal stent placement may reduce recurrent stenosis and/or serve as an adjunct to balloon dilation.

Video 9.15 Flexible bronchoscopy demonstrating a distal tracheal rupture with extension into the mediastinum.

TRACHEOPATHIES

Tracheopathies encompass a broad spectrum of disease processes, a subset of which will be discussed here. These may occur in the setting of mucopolysaccharidoses (e.g., Hunter's or Hurler's syndromes), cartilage abnormalities in the setting of specific syndromes (e.g., Apert, Crouzon, Pfieffer syndromes), and those that accompany some cardiovascular defects (e.g., left pulmonary artery sling), to name but a few. Airway management may require a multitude of endoscopic techniques, including those associated with facial skeletal abnormalities or laryngeal and pharyngeal pathology. Additionally, central airway anomalies, spinal anomalies, and restrictive thoracic pathology may exist.

MUCOPOLYSACCHARIDOSES (MPS)

- **Upper airway pathology**
  - The accumulation of glycosaminoglycans in the oropharynx and larynx may lead to difficulty ventilating and/or intubating a child. A variety of bronchoscopic techniques exist to assist in this setting.
  - An awake flexible transnasal laryngoscopy may provide useful information with regard to the appearance of the larynx and surrounding soft tissues. It should be understood that, once anesthetized, the airway will always prove more difficult to visualize. As a general rule-of-thumb for MPS patients, the airway that appears easy to intubate will be difficult, and the airway that appears difficult to intubate may be nearly impossible.
  - Placement of a laryngeal mask airway (LMA) or oropharyngeal airway prior to flexible endoscopic intubation may allow for improved ventilation. If ventilation is adequate with an LMA, flexible bronchoscopy through the LMA may be attempted. Unfortunately, under many circumstances, these adjuncts are not successful in maintaining a patent airway and one must be prepared to use alternative techniques to establish the airway (Video 9.16).
  - Direct laryngoscopy with intubation over a Hopkins rod or with a rigid bronchoscope may be successful in less severe disease.
  - Hybrid approaches, using a videolaryngoscope and flexible bronchoscope may provide the visualization necessary to achieve flexible bronchoscopic intubation.
  - Under all circumstances, one must be prepared to perform a tracheostomy.
- **Central and lower airway pathology**
  - Restrictive lung disease may result as a consequence of diaphragmatic motion limitation or due to anatomic abnormalities of the thorax. This may result in reduced excursion and compound tracheal abnormalities visualized by bronchoscopy. Taking these factors into consideration during bronchoscopy is important, as this pathology visualized during the procedure may influence the decision making.
  - Significant soft-tissue redundancy and tracheal wall thickening due to MPS deposits frequently lead to progressive tracheomalacia and bronchomalacia. Flexible bronchoscopy is ideally poised to diagnose and track these processes, as it can be performed under less sedation or through a tracheostomy tube when present (Video 9.17).
  - Examination for mucosal injuries in the setting of tracheostomy tube placement should always be performed during endoscopic evaluation. Withdrawing the tracheostomy tube to visualize the mucosa at the location of the tracheostomy tube is important, particularly if there is any history of bleeding from the airway.
  - Avoiding placement of the tracheostomy tube tip at the location of the innominate artery, especially in patients with severe malacia, is prudent. This may require a customized tracheostomy tube, or adjustments to the length of the tube over time.

Video 9.16 Severe glossoptosis, and epiglottic prolapse in a patient with mucopolysaccharidosis.

Video 9.17 Flexible bronchoscopy demonstrating moderate to severe tracheomalacia and airway deposits in a patient with mucopolysaccharidosis.

SELECT TRACHEAL CARTILAGE ABNORMALITIES

- **Congenital tracheal stenosis: Complete tracheal rings**
  - Rigid bronchoscopy is the criterion standard diagnostic modality for tracheal stenosis.
  - Flexible bronchoscopy is also frequently performed; however, this is most often done primarily to assess the lower airway and pulmonary anatomy.
  - During all bronchoscopic procedures, caution must be exercised to reduce airway inflammation at the level of the stenotic segment.
  - Rigid bronchoscopy provides improved optics and tactile feedback and allows the practitioner to visualize and size the airway safely, with a few important considerations in mind:
    - Congenital tracheal stenosis frequently becomes more severe as one travels inferiorly through the airway. The practitioner must anticipate this progressive narrowing and avoid contacting the mucosa circumferentially or "forcing" a scope through the stenotic segment (Video 9.18). There should always be space around the endoscope during the procedure. The size of a conventional rigid telescope should be selected based on the size of the airway lumen. If unknown, the narrowest available endoscope should be selected.
    - Sizing the airway can be accomplished using conventional ETTs, although the trachea may be too narrow for this option. "Leading" the rigid endoscope with a small suction catheter allows for direct visualization of the airway lumen, with the catheter present for reference. It is not uncommon for patients with tracheal stenosis to have an airway that "cones" down to the outer diameter of a 5F–8F catheter (Video 9.19).
    - If intubation is required, the tube can be placed while simultaneously visualizing the airway through the tube with an endoscope, placing it immediately above the stenosis or in a wider, proximal segment.
    - If the ETT must be placed within the proximal ring segment, choose an atraumatic tube size and visualize through the sidewall of the ETT for evidence of blanching. If blanching is present, downsize or withdraw the tube, if possible.
    - Avoid placing a cuffed ETT when feasible. If there is ample room above the stenotic segment to place an ETT and the cuff is required to achieve adequate ventilation, mark the position of the ETT while directly visualizing the tube position endoscopically. Avoid tube mobility until extubation.
    - Small volumes of vasoconstricting or anti-inflammatory medications may be used in the setting of airway inflammation. This may include epinephrine or dexamethasone drops *via* the ETT or in a nebulized fashion.
    - Repositioning of the ETT, if present, should be done under bronchoscopic guidance where appropriate.
- **Tracheal cartilaginous sleeve (TCS)**
  - Should be suspected in patients with Apert, Crouzon, and Pfeiffer syndromes, among others.
  - This airway malformation involves a continuous segment of cartilage forming a segment of the trachea rather than tracheal rings.
  - The segment is often stenotic, and may involve all or part of the trachea, and/or mainstem bronchi.

- Endoscopic evaluation can be performed using rigid or flexible bronchoscopy. Sizing the airway should be performed using rigid techniques, and care should be taken to avoid airway trauma or mucosal inflammation, including intubation with an ETT that is larger than the airway lumen.
- Flexible bronchoscopy allows for visualization of the involved segment as well as clearance of distal airway secretions.
- Attempts at balloon dilation should be avoided.
- Patients frequently have systemic, multi-organ involvement, and consideration of anesthetic technique and patient stability must be considered prior to and during bronchoscopy.
- Surgical intervention may be required in a subset of patients.

Video 9.18 Severe airway inflammation in a patient with complete tracheal rings. In this video, the telescope is pushed through the ring segment after meeting some resistance. This is an example of what *not* to do in this setting.

Video 9.19 Rigid bronchoscopy demonstrating a patient with long-segment complete tracheal rings. A 5 French suction catheter is present in the lumen. The distal airway narrows to a caliber that is just large enough to accommodate the catheter.

WHOLE-LUNG LAVAGE

INDICATIONS

Whole-lung lavage (WLL) or large-volume lung lavage is the primary treatment for certain forms of pulmonary alveolar proteinosis (PAP). It is also used to treat other alveolar-filling diseases such as lipoid pneumonia. PAP is a rare condition with accumulation of phospholipoproteinaceous material in the alveoli which impairs gas exchange, leading to respiratory insufficiency and hypoxic respiratory failure. Disturbance in surfactant homeostasis is caused by abnormal surfactant production, processing, and/or removal. Often, the lung is affected diffusely, with computed tomography (CT) of the chest showing ground glass opacities and interlobular and intralobular septal thickening. WLL attempts to clear this proteinaceous material, resulting in improvement of symptoms. Patients who are symptomatic and/or have impaired activities of daily life and/or have failure to thrive may be considered for WLL. The challenge of this intervention lies within the balance of providing respiratory support of the patient while administering lavage fluid to wash the affected lung at the same time. The approach is selective isolation of a single lung for washing and providing ventilation *via* the trachea to the contralateral lung. PAP can be primary or secondary. Patients may need repeated sessions of intervention to result in clinical improvement. The intervention may need to be repeated if the proteinaceous material re-accumulates.

PREPARATION

- **Patient factors**
  - *Affected areas*: PAP is usually diffuse, though peripheral and dependent areas may be more affected. Chest imaging with chest CT is helpful to identify areas to target for lavage. Post-intervention chest imaging can show improvement of the ground glass opacities seen in PAP.
  - *Patient age and weight*: The patient's age and weight defines the equipment that can be used for simultaneous whole-lung wash and single-lung ventilation. WLL was initially described in adults[2,3] and utilized double-lumen ETTs to selectively isolate a lung for large-volume washing. The smallest double-lumen ETT is 26 French (approximately 8.7 mm). For small patients or children < 8 years, there are alternative approaches for single-lung ventilation and access to the contralateral lung for WLL. Techniques include using cuffed ETTs[4] or balloon catheters.[5,6] An alternative method is to perform selective lobar lavages.[7]

- For patients > 8 years, utilize double-lumen ETT.
- For 1- to 8-year-old patients, use an ETT and a second cuffed ETT or an extra-long croup tube or Foley catheter as the bronchial tube.
- For <1-year-old patients, use cuffed ETTs and a pulmonary artery catheter.
   - *Patient stability*: For WLL, the patient needs to be able to tolerate single-lung ventilation. Often, the healthier lung is chosen for isolated ventilation while the more diseased lung is lavaged. If a patient is unable to tolerate single-lung ventilation, then segmental bronchoalveolar washing can be pursued.
   - WLL can also be done while the patient is supported with extra-corporeal membrane oxygenation, if necessary.
- **Equipment**
   - *Double-lumen ETTs*: The smallest double-lumen ETT is 26 French (8.7 mm). The youngest average-sized patient for this ETT is 8 years old.
   - *Alternative bronchial tubes*
      - Cuffed ETTs: Small cuffed ETTs can be placed in a bronchus to selectively isolate a lung. Tube connectors may need to be used to elongate the tube to allow for proper placement in the bronchus and instillation and drainage of fluid. Often the ETT is placed transnasally to better secure it and minimize risk of movement during the procedure.
      - Pulmonary artery catheter:[5,6] 4–8 French, external diameter ranges from 1.35 to 2.7 mm.
      - Foley urinary catheter[8] 16 French = 5.28 mm external diameter
   - *Lavage fluid*
      - Warmed fluid: Normal saline heated to 36–37°C. Warming can be done by a combination of a bath, inline heat exchanger, and radiant warmers.
      - Size of the aliquot has been varied from standard aliquots in adults at 500–1000 mL,[5,9] based on pre-operative measurement of functional residual capacity (FRC),[10] (5–10 mL/kg),[4] 20 mL/kg.[5]
      - Infusion of lavage fluid: Manual by hand or gravity *versus* automated with infusion pumps. Infusion by gravity allows the infusion pressure to be set based on the height of the bag of saline above the lung being lavaged (typically ~ 30 cm) and the infusion volume to be regulated accordingly. This also lessens the risk of leaks since there is less variability in infusion pressure. Caution must be taken when infusing by hand or when using automated infusion pumps due to the risk of barotrauma by instilling fluid under pressure. resulting in pneumohydrothorax.
      - **Figure 9.7** demonstrates the key features of one possible setup.
   - *Chest physiotherapy*: Manual or mechanical[11] chest percussion can be done during the procedure to promote mobilization of the proteinaceous material.
   - *Table setup*: Allow space to line up aliquots of effluent to track the improvement of sediment in the fluid over time (**Figure 9.8**).

PERFORMING THE PROCEDURE

- Patient preparation is achieved with temperature regulation using a heated blanket and mattress. Patient can be supine or in a full or partial lateral decubitus position with the lung undergoing treatment in the superior position if the lungs are effectively isolated. Full[12] or partial[11] lateral decubitus with the treatment lung up can help maximize the drainage of the effluent and improve ventilation-perfusion matching of the dependent lung that is being ventilated. If unable to isolate the lungs and carrying out segmental lung lavage, then placing the lung being targeted for lavage in the dependent position may reduce the spill-over of fluid into the contralateral lung.
- Insertion of a double-lumen ETT or insertion of a bronchial tube for lung isolation, followed by insertion of age-appropriate endotracheal or contralateral bronchial tube for ventilation.[8]
   - Insertion of alternative catheters, such as a pulmonary artery catheter, can be done within the lumen of the tracheal tube.[6]
   - Proper catheter position is verified by flexible bronchoscopy.

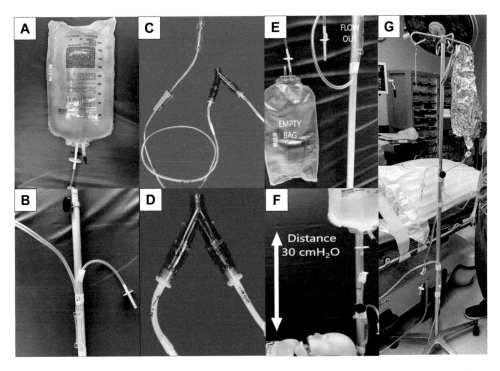

Figure 9.7 Whole-lung lavage setup utilizing two bladder irrigation kits and an IV pole. (A) 3-L bag of normal saline attached to (B) bladder irrigation kit with chamber to allow visualization of saline flow. (C) Flow regulator attached to tubing and connected to (D) Y-adaptor with inflow and outflow lines labeled. (E) Second bladder irrigation kit draining effluent to the ground. (F) Inflow bag is placed approximately 30 cm above the patient's chest to regulate filling pressure. (G) The entire setup is assembled in the OR with aluminum foil covering the saline bag to better maintain temperature.

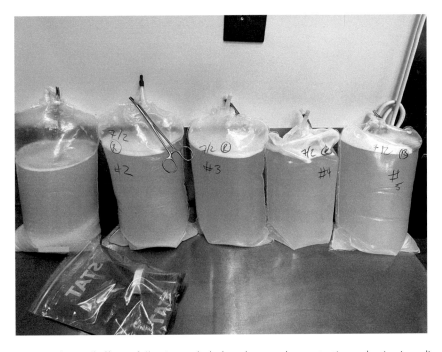

Figure 9.8 Five 3-L bags of effluent following a whole-lung lavage, demonstrating reduction in sediment during the procedure.

- Inflation of cuffs to ensure lung isolation and ventilation without leak. Endotracheal or endobronchial tube used for ventilation can be without cuff if adequate ventilation can be maintained.
- Ventilation with 100% oxygen is provided to both the bronchial tube and the tracheal tube.
- Proper tube position is verified by flexible bronchoscopy.[13]
- Lung isolation is verified by providing selective ventilation and auscultation.
- Test lavage with 1 mL/kg bodyweight is done in the bronchial tube with bronchoscopic visualization through the tracheal tube to ensure that there is no leakage from the bronchus/lung undergoing treatment.
- Discontinue ventilation and connect to saline administration system.
- Instill warmed saline into the bronchial tube by gravity or gentle pressure with 50 mL syringe.
  - The volume of saline can be estimated based on pre-operative FRC or can be weight based, such as 5–20 mL/kg.
  - Instillation by gravity allows the volume instilled to be regulated by the height of the saline bag above the lung being lavaged (typically ~ 30 cm). Fluid is instilled until the flow stops.
  - Chest physiotherapy can be done once the fluid is instilled to encourage the mobilization of proteinaceous material.
  - Manual percussion has been shown to be superior to mechanical percussion or no percussion in one study.[14]
- Effluent fluid is drained from the bronchial tube by gravity. No dwell time is recommended due to concerns for systemic absorption and prolonging the procedure.
- Lavage is repeated until the appearance of the effluent fluid is clear with minimal sediment (**Figure 9.9**).[15,16]
  - Intra-operative measurement of optical density (OD), using a spectrometer, has been described.[5] Lavage is discontinued once the OD is < 0.4.
- The remaining fluid can be aspirated by flexible bronchoscopy, but this isn't always needed.
- Ventilation to the bronchial tube is resumed initially with bag ventilation to re-recruit the lung.
- The bronchial tube is removed.
- The ETT is now ventilated to allow double-lung ventilation.

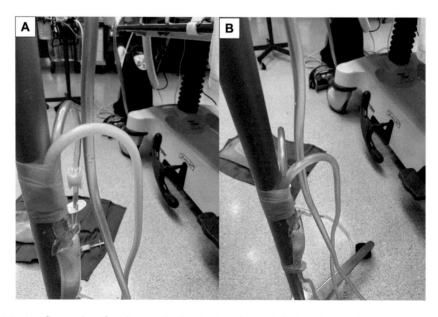

Figure 9.9 (A) Inflow and outflow lines at the beginning of the whole-lung lavage demonstrating significant sediment removal. (B) Inflow and outflow lines at the conclusion of the whole-lung lavage, demonstrating marked improvement.

PRECAUTIONS

- Hypoxemia often occurs during the procedure due to VQ mismatch. During draining of the effluent, the airway pressure decreases in the lung undergoing treatment, which can cause pulmonary blood to flow to the impaired lung and result in a fall in PaO_2.
- Loss of lung isolation will result in overspill of the lavage fluid into the ventilated lung. If lavage fluid is seen in the tracheal tube, the lavage can be stopped. Flexible bronchoscopy through the tracheal tube should be performed to confirm and adjust the bronchial tube.
- Dislodgement of the bronchial tube can occur.
- Vocal cord edema or subglottic trauma can occurs resulting from the need to fit large-caliber tubes in a pediatric airway. Treatment is with peri-extubation steroids.
- Complications must be reported: e.g., pleural effusion, hydropneumothorax, hypothermia.

FOLLOWING THE PROCEDURE

- Post-procedure lung volume recruitment should continue.
- Extubation: Mechanical ventilation can be continued for as long as needed for lung recruitment before extubation, but a prolonged time is not always necessary.
- Some patients are able to be safely extubated in the OR and discharged home the same day in select instances.
- If necessary, post-procedural care should take place in a unit equipped to support mechanical ventilation, with respiratory therapists for endotracheal suctioning, to facilitate extubation, provide post-extubation respiratory support, and possibly re-intubation.

PLASTIC BRONCHITIS

Plastic bronchitis is a condition leading to formed branching casts filling the airways (Figure 9.10). It is associated with cardiac abnormalities, cystic fibrosis, asthma, sickle cell anemia, lymphagiomatosis, and can occur idiopathically. It is most commonly seen in patients with single-ventricle heart disease after palliation.

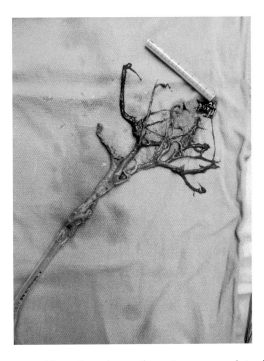

Figure 9.10 Bronchial cast removed from airway by gentle suction on an endotracheal tube.

The casts can be made up of protein, fibrin, mucin, or inflammatory cells. Obstruction of the airway leads to hypoxemia, cough, and respiratory distress. Treatment includes bronchoscopy for cast removal and medical management with inhaled medications and chest physiotherapy.[17]

ENDOSCOPIC MANAGEMENT

Either flexible bronchoscopy or rigid bronchoscopy can be utilized to remove casts. The casts can be friable or tenacious, with many segmental branches leading to long roots. Removal can be done with suction, dislodgement with saline or mucolytics, or forceps. Direct airway instillation of tissue plasminogen activator (tPA) can be used to break up fibrin.

- tPA 0.5 mg/mL solution, 1-mL aliquots for instillation.[18]

MEDICAL MANAGEMENT

Inhaled medications, such as tPA, dornase, or hypertonic saline, delivered by nebulization can help break up the casts. Chest physiotherapy is also utilized to dislodge cast, allowing patients to expectorate the cast. Inhaled steroids, antibiotics, and systemic steroids have been utilized as treatment if there is an inflammatory process involved in cast formation.

- tPA 1 mg/mL solution, 5 mg nebulized every 2–8 hours with a maximum dose of 1 mg/kg/day for a limited course, 1–14 days.[18–21] Long-term treatment can involve 5 mg nebulized up to every 6 hours.[22] There is a risk of pulmonary hemorrhage.

Surgical approaches to optimize Fontan physiology in single-ventricle heart patients can reduce cast formation. Lymphatic abnormalities can also lead to cast formation so these can be treated with thoracic duct ligation.

CONCLUSION AND TIPS FOR CLINICAL PRACTICE

It behooves the astute practitioner to learn techniques, instruments, and skillsets that may not be a core facet of their specialty training. Airway specialists with training in rigid endoscopy should learn the nuances of flexible bronchoscopy and vice-versa. Moreover, adult and pediatric endoscopists should be aware of the differences between adult and pediatric physiology, anesthetic techniques, and pathologic processes that apply to each population. Much can be learned from those around us who do things in a different way, and an open mind is often the most essential requirement in solving a complex or unique problem affecting the airway.

Teamwork is key during bronchoscopy for specific indications in pediatrics. This chapter describes some rare conditions and specific procedures which may be rarely done. Preparation and communication is of utmost importance. All the personnel present during the procedure will need to be engaged and participate to result in a successful procedure.

REFERENCES

1. Park JA, Kim BJ. Intrapulmonary recombinant factor VIIa for diffuse alveolar hemorrhage in children. *Pediatrics.* 2015;135(1):e216–20.
2. Ramirez J, Schultz RB, Dutton RE. Pulmonary alveolar proteinosis: a new technique and rationale for treatment. *Arch Intern Med.* 1963;112:419–31.
3. Ramirez J, Kieffer RF, Jr., Ball WC, Jr. Bronchopulmonary lavage in man. *Ann Intern Med.* 1965;63(5):819–28.
4. Paquet C, Karsli C. Technique of lung isolation for whole lung lavage in a child with pulmonary alveolar proteinosis. *Anesthesiology.* 2009;110(1):190–2.
5. Paschen C, Reiter K, Stanzel F, Teschler H, Griese M. Therapeutic lung lavages in children and adults. *Respir Res.* 2005;6:138.

6. Reiter K, Schoen C, Griese M, Nicolai T. Whole-lung lavage in infants and children with pulmonary alveolar proteinosis. *Paediatr Anaesth.* 2010;20(12):1118–23.

7. de Blic J. Pulmonary alveolar proteinosis in children. *Paediatr Respir Rev.* 2004;5(4):316–22.

8. Wilson CA, Wilmshurst SL, Black AE. Anesthetic techniques to facilitate lung lavage for pulmonary alveolar proteinosis in children-new airway techniques and a review of the literature. *Paediatr Anaesth.* 2015;25(6):546–53.

9. Abdelmalak BB, Khanna AK, Culver DA, Popovich MJ. Therapeutic whole-lung lavage for pulmonary alveolar proteinosis: a procedural update. *J Bronchology Interv Pulmonol.* 2015;22(3):251–8.

10. Shah PL, Hansell D, Lawson PR, Reid KB, Morgan C. Pulmonary alveolar proteinosis: clinical aspects and current concepts on pathogenesis. *Thorax.* 2000;55(1):67–77.

11. Moy EK, Pistun O, Teba C, Jagpal S, Hussain S. A rapid infuser system for whole-lung lavage. *J Bronchology Interv Pulmonol.* 2016;23(1):e6–8.

12. Alasiri AM, Alasbali RA, Alaqil MA, Alahmari AM, Alshamrani ND, Badri RN. Autoimmune pulmonary alveolar proteinosis successfully treated with lung lavage in an adolescent patient: a case report. *J Med Case Rep.* 2021;15(1):340.

13. Sigakis MJG, De Cardenas JL. Lung ultrasound scans during whole lung lavage. *Chest.* 2021;159(6):e433–e6.

14. Hammon WE, McCaffree DR, Cucchiara AJ. A comparison of manual to mechanical chest percussion for clearance of alveolar material in patients with pulmonary alveolar proteinosis (phospholipidosis). *Chest.* 1993;103(5):1409–12.

15. Bingisser R, Kaplan V, Zollinger A, Russi EW. Whole-lung lavage in alveolar proteinosis by a modified lavage technique. *Chest.* 1998;113(6):1718–9.

16. Bonella F, Bauer PC, Griese M, Wessendorf TE, Guzman J, Costabel U. Wash-out kinetics and efficacy of a modified lavage technique for alveolar proteinosis. *Eur Respir J.* 2012;40(6):1468–74.

17. Li Y, Williams RJ, Dombrowski ND, Watters K, Daly KP, Irace AL, et al. Current evaluation and management of plastic bronchitis in the pediatric population. *Int J Pediatr Otorhinolaryngol.* 2020;130:109799.

18. Gibb E, Blount R, Lewis N, Nielson D, Church G, Jones K, et al. Management of plastic bronchitis with topical tissue-type plasminogen activator. *Pediatrics.* 2012;130(2):e446–50.

19. Costello JM, Steinhorn D, McColley S, Gerber ME, Kumar SP. Treatment of plastic bronchitis in a Fontan patient with tissue plasminogen activator: a case report and review of the literature. *Pediatrics.* 2002;109(4):e67.

20. Do T, Chu JM, Farhouch B, Anas N. Fontan patient with plastic bronchitis treated successfully using aerosolized tissue plasminogen activator. *Pediatr Cardiol.* 2009;30:352–5.

21. Lubcke NL, Nussbaum VM, Schroth M. Use of aerosolized tissue plasminogen activator in the treatment of plastic bronchitis. *Ann Pharmacother.* 2013;47(3):e13.

22. Wakeham MK, Van Bergen AH, Torero LE, Akhter J. Long-term treatment of plastic bronchitis with aerosolized tissue plasminogen activator in a Fontan patient. *Pediatr Crit Care Med.* 2005;6(1):76–8.

10

Bronchoscopy training and simulation for medical education

RIDDHIMA AGARWAL, EMILY DeBOER, AND TENDY CHIANG

INTRODUCTION

Program directors across multiple pediatric specialties, including pulmonology, otolaryngology, and general surgery, have critically discussed trainee preparedness in performing both rigid and flexible bronchoscopy.[1–5] Bronchoscopy is a complex, psychomotor skill that is best developed with volume and repetition. Unfortunately, pediatric providers are notably limited by a lack of exposure to this technique during residency and fellowship training, especially in emergency settings. Indeed, it has been estimated that otolaryngology residents and pediatric surgery fellows participate in as few as 1–2 foreign body removals per year.[6,7] Meanwhile, the number of flexible bronchoscopies performed by pediatric pulmonology fellows during a 3-year program can range broadly from 10 to 200.[8]

Given the scarcity of cases requiring pediatric rigid bronchoscopy, specifically cases that include intervention, the traditional "see one, do one, teach one" apprenticeship model does not provide trainees with reliable, structured, and standardized opportunities for learning. Moreover, the use of this approach to teaching a high-stakes, invasive procedure can place patients at an unjustifiable risk of complications and suboptimal outcomes.[9,10]

Development of a procedural skill can be divided into two phases. During an initial cognitive phase, learners acquire theoretical background knowledge. The subsequent psychomotor phase provides hands-on practical experience, first *via* simulation and then on patients under graduated supervision.[10,11] "Competency" requires (1) mastering cognitive knowledge about the procedure, including the unique anatomy of the pediatric airway, (2) acquiring technical skills, (3) combining the above in order to perform procedures safely, (4) obtaining accurate diagnostic information, (5) interacting cooperatively with an interdisciplinary team, and (6) troubleshooting unusual circumstances.

Although they assess similar anatomy, rigid and flexible bronchoscopy are distinct skills with different goals. Given that the training philosophy for both are similar, in this chapter, we have purposely used the term "bronchoscopy" where statements apply to either procedure. It is important to remember that trainees from medical *versus* surgical subspecialties have different clinical training experiences and cultures. Although innate differences in 3-dimensional spatial reasoning have not been observed between these two groups,[12] it is important to consider individual differences across your learners.

This chapter begins by describing key learning points, modes of instruction, and teaching philosophies within each phase of training/learning. Subsequent sections explain accreditation requirements and tools for ascertaining competency, both during training and as a part of continued professional development. We conclude by highlighting future opportunities in pediatric bronchoscopy education.

TEACHING METHODS

COGNITIVE PHASE OF PEDIATRIC BRONCHOSCOPY TRAINING

There is a growing body of literature stating the importance of deconstructing complex psychomotor tasks, such as bronchoscopy, into their component parts.[13] Although medical, technical, and clinical knowledge may be taught (or learned) concurrently, it is important that the teacher considers this breakdown (Table 10.1) in their bronchoscopy curriculum and ensures that each trainee receives mastery in all three categories.[10,14]

MEDICAL KNOWLEDGE – ANATOMY AND PHYSIOLOGY OF THE PEDIATRIC AIRWAY

Pediatric airway anatomy differs in many ways from its adult counterpart, thereby creating distinct challenges for airway assessment and stabilization (Table 10.2). For example, visualization of the pediatric airway *via* direct laryngoscopy is impeded by larger oropharyngeal structures and more cephalad position of the larynx. Additionally, anatomic differences in the occiput and epiglottis must be considered when positioning a patient and selecting instrumentation. Lastly, multiple anatomic structures, particularly the shorter and narrower trachea, predispose children to airway obstruction.[15] These differences are important to highlight during the initial phases of education.

Pediatric patients have physiological challenges that increase their risk of respiratory failure with rapid desaturation. Children have shorter, safe apneic intervals than adults due to lower functional residual capacity and faster rates of oxygen metabolism. Additionally, pediatric patients are readily susceptible to respiratory fatigue because they have a lower percentage of energy-efficient, slow-twitch skeletal muscle fibers within their intercostal muscles and diaphragm. The susceptibility for respiratory fatigue is intensified by the need for intrinsic muscles to maintain lung volumes in the setting of higher chest wall compliance.[15]

When evaluating a pediatric patient, it is also crucial to assess for common syndromes and congenital anomalies that are associated with difficult airway management.[16] Education should include hands-on examples for common diagnoses, such as trisomy 21, as well as written and generalized examples for rarer, but uniquely important conditions (Table 10.3).

Table 10.1 Theoretical foundation for pediatric bronchoscopy

Medical knowledge	• Understand pediatric airway anatomy and physiology
Technical and instrument knowledge	• Understand the scope of endoscopic interventions used in diagnosing and treating various airway pathologies • Assemble, appropriately use, and maintain associated equipment • Know procedural steps
Clinical knowledge	• Accurately and comprehensively evaluate the patient, including pre-operative and intra-operative interpretation of diagnostic findings • Identify risks and benefits of the procedure, as well as optimizing pre-operative health • Develop an anesthesia and airway plan • Recognize, prevent, manage, and monitor for possible complications

Table 10.2 Clinical implications of pediatric airway anatomy

Structure	Pediatric feature (as compared with adults)	Significance
Occiput	Proportionally larger, resulting in neck flexion while supine	• Impaired visualization of glottic opening during laryngoscopy • Potential for airway obstruction (airway alignment can be improved by placing a towel roll beneath the shoulders)
Tongue	Larger relative to oral cavity size	• Impaired visualization of deeper airway during laryngoscopy • Increased risk of retroglossal obstruction
Lymphoid tissue	Increased mass Risk of adenoidal bleeding from naso-tracheal/pharyngeal intubation	• Source of airway obstruction • Aspiration risk
Larynx	Located opposite C3 and C4 vertebrae (compared with C4 and C5 in adults)	• Impaired visualization during laryngoscopy
Epiglottis	Larger; more acutely angled relative to the trachea; Lower tensile strength of hyoepiglottic ligament	• Curved blades are less effective at elevating epiglottis (improved mobilization with a straight blade)
Trachea	Shorter	• Increased risk of right mainstem bronchus intubation or accidental extubation
	Narrower	• According to Poiseuille's Law, airway resistance is inversely proportional to the luminal radius raised to the 4th power. Thus, similar decreases in airway diameter (as a result of edema, secretions, stenosis, or compression) will more significantly increase airway resistance in a smaller *versus* a larger airway
	Smaller cricothyroid membrane	• Cricothyroidotomy is more challenging
Subglottis	Narrowest portion of airway (compared with glottis in adults)	• Foreign bodies are more likely to lodge below the vocal cords

Table 10.3 Features and etiologies of complicated pediatric airways

Predictor of difficult airway	Associated condition
Dysmorphic features	• Mucopolysaccharidoses
Restricted neck mobility	• Trisomy 21
	• Mucopolysaccharidoses
Nasopharyngeal obstruction	• Choanal atresia (CHARGE syndrome)
Abnormal jaw anatomy	**Mandibular hypoplasia**
	• Trisomy 21
	• Pierre Robin sequence
	• Treacher Collins syndrome
	• Mucopolysaccharidoses
	Maxillary hypoplasia
	• Beckwith-Wiedemann syndrome
	• Treacher Collins syndrome
	Other
	• Pierre Robin sequence: Micrognathia and retrognathia
	• Treacher Collins syndrome: Zygomatic hypoplasia
Restricted temporomandibular joint mobility	• Treacher Collins syndrome
	• Mucopolysaccharidoses
Abnormal tongue anatomy	**Macroglossia**
	• Trisomy 21
	• Beckwith-Wiedemann syndrome
	• Mucopolysaccharidoses
	Glossoptosis
	• Pierre Robin sequence
Tonsillar and adenoid hypertrophy	• Trisomy 21
	• Mucopolysaccharidoses
Structurally abnormal laryngeal passage	• Laryngomalacia
	• Laryngeal webs
	• Congenital or acquired subglottic stenosis
Structurally abnormal tracheal passage	• Tracheobronchomalacia
	• Tracheoesophageal fistula
	• Vascular ring
	• Congenital or acquired tracheal stenosis
Other	• Beckwith-Wiedemann syndrome: Visceromegaly shifts diaphragm upward, thereby decreasing functional residual capacity

TECHNICAL, INSTRUMENTAL, AND CLINICAL KNOWLEDGE

Learners should have a foundational understanding of the technical, instrumental, and clinical considerations within pediatric bronchoscopy before seeking practical experience with the technique.[14] Chapters 1 and 2 of this text review pediatric bronchoscopy indications, and contraindications. Chapter 2 also explains pre- and post-operative management for pediatric bronchoscopy and compares flexible *versus* rigid techniques. Equipment and interventional techniques (thermal and non-thermal) are detailed in Chapters 2, 3, and 8, respectively. Lastly, operative techniques are described in Chapters 6 and 7. As teachers, it is important to help learners integrate this textbook knowledge with clinical practice and hands-on learning.

MODES OF DELIVERING THEORETICAL KNOWLEDGE

The traditional lecture-based method of classroom instruction presumes that all participants are at the same stage of training, relies on passive learning, and offers minimal opportunities for teachers and students to exchange feedback. Alternative, student-centered instructional methods have increasingly been applied to medical education, including pediatric bronchoscopy training.[11] Web-based resources, including online courses, society websites, electronic books, podcasts, apps, and teleconferences, provide scalable, up-to-date content. The inherent advantage of E-learning is the flexibility and personalization it offers.[9,10] The Bronchoscopy International website, for example, is a free, online resource that provides two series, "The Essential Bronchoscopist" and "BronchAtlas", covering the fundamentals of bronchoscopy.[17]

Perhaps the ideal use of web-based resources is in the setting of flipped classroom instruction. *Via* this method, students review content independently, leaving classroom time to clarify questions and participate in Problem-Based Learning (PBL). The "Four-Box Practical Approach to Interventional Bronchoscopy"[17] is a type of PBL that includes a series of case studies, testing (1) pre-procedure evaluation, (2) procedural techniques, (3) strategies based on expected and unexpected intra-operative findings, and (4) short- *versus* long-term follow-up. A trainee's depth of understanding is judged based on their ability to justify rationale using current literature, experimental data, and clinical experience. Learners are therefore given the opportunity to both demonstrate cognitive knowledge and to practice evidence-based clinical decision making. Journal clubs and grand rounds are less structured, but adjunctive tools for delivering information in a focused area of interest or research.[9,10]

PRACTICAL TRAINING FOR PEDIATRIC BRONCHOSCOPY – CURRENT STATE OF SIMULATION

BRONCHOSCOPY SIMULATORS

Simulation-based procedural training offers safe, low-stakes, and controlled opportunities to apply technical and instrumental knowledge, as well as to practice associated non-technical skills.[18] Historically, pediatric airway simulation dates as far back as the late 1800s when Dr. Chevalier Jackson, known as the "Father of Bronchoesophagoscopy", demonstrated endoscopic foreign body retrieval on "Michelle the Choking Doll".[19]

At present, the majority of simulation technology is designed to instruct in adult, flexible bronchoscopy.[18] Currently available simulators for pediatric rigid bronchoscopy are physical, directly manipulable models into which standard bronchoscopes can be introduced. These can be categorized by fidelity, which refers to the realism of the simulator itself or the environment in which it is used. Both low- and high-fidelity physical models allow trainees to improve hand–eye coordination and build muscle memory with traditional operative equipment.[10,20,21]

High-fidelity mannequins can be programmed to (1) depict anatomic anomalies, (2) produce physiologic response (e.g., cardio-respiratory movements, coughing) or resistance to scope insertion, (3) recreate associated complications (e.g., desaturation or iatrogenic bleeding), and (4) monitor and grade trainee performance. A notable advantage of high-fidelity video simulators with feedback is that they consolidate all phases of learning and allow the practice of rare cases, anatomy, and airway emergencies. Limitations of high-fidelity video simulators include cost and fragility of equipment, as well as scheduling constraints within a simulation studio. Low-fidelity anatomy simulators have fewer barriers to cost and scheduling, but can often only educate on medical knowledge, anatomy, and basic technical skills. Combining multiple types of lectures, simulation, and apprenticeship can maximize the learning experience.[10,20,21]

Ram et al.[22] developed a porcine model that resembled the respiratory tract of an 8- to 12-year-old child and allowed use of a 7.0 ventilating bronchoscope. Although a porcine tracheobronchial tree mimics the tissue quality and compliance of a human airway more realistically than does synthetic material, its many structural differences include a longer epiglottis, a more anteriorly positioned larynx, and less prominent tracheal rings.[22] Use of cadaveric parts is further limited by ethical concerns, cost of animal care resources, and limited shelf-life.[10]

Jabbour et al.[13] designed a simulation-based pediatric airway endoscopy course in which participants performed rigid bronchoscopy on a Laerdal Neonatal Intubation Trainer (low-fidelity), followed by foreign body retrieval on a SimNewB Neonatal Simulator and organosilicate analog model of the airway of a 7-year-old patient. Though the SimNewB Neonatal Simulator is a high-fidelity mannequin, it was used in passive mode. The 3-dimensionally (3D)-printed replica was created using computed tomography and magnetic resonance imaging scans of multiple patients with normal anatomy. Although these replicas could be used for flexible bronchoscopy, they needed to be covered with the "skin" of commercially available mannequins for use with rigid bronchoscopes.[13]

Multiple groups have since digitally reconstructed and 3D-printed pediatric airway models. Although the replica of an 18-month-old tracheobronchial tree by Hsiung et al. used a rubber-plastic composite that was more amenable to rigid bronchoscopy for foreign body retrieval, this model had size constraints related to its manufacturing process.[6] Al-Ramahi et al.[23] successfully created a scalable model using a rubber-like material. To mimic the developing mechanical properties of the human trachea, the stiffness of the material was adjusted according to the desired age group. Use of synthetic material limited both groups' ability to replicate respiratory mucosa, airway secretions, and tracheal rings.[23] DeBoer et al. found that novice learners significantly improved in terms of bronchial anatomy knowledge and flexible bronchoscope manipulation with less than 1 hour of practice and only 15 minutes of directed teaching using a 3D-printed anatomy trainer.[24]

Deutsch et al.[25] and Griffin et al.[26] described rigid bronchoscopy on high-fidelity, computerized infant mannequins, programmed to simulate endobronchial foreign body lodgment. Participants across the two studies recognized and responded to changes in the simulated patient's condition, including worsening stridor, asymmetric chest wall motion, desaturation, and laryngospasm.[25,26]

PRACTICING NON-TECHNICAL SKILLS

It has repeatedly been reported that medical errors occur more commonly due to failure in non-technical skills rather than to a lack of technical expertise. Although non-technical skills have been classified in multiple ways, a common approach considers four broad categories: communication, teamwork, leadership, and decision making.[11]

Frequently identified sources of surgical errors in particular include (1) lack of communication between the surgical and anesthesiology team, (2) failure to anticipate or prepare for unplanned events, and (3) lack of pre-operative briefing or post-operative debriefing.[10] Educators should demonstrate excellent non-technical skills and purposely reflect upon the steps their learners can take to prevent non-technical lapses during pediatric bronchoscopy.

Shared operating rooms (OR) can be noisy environments where the use of face coverings, especially N-95s and similar respirators, obstructs auditory and visual cues. Thus, communication between the bronchoscopist, anesthesiologist, and OR team should begin outside of the OR. In addition to a surgical time-out, careful discussion of the planned and unplanned operative course will ensure that all teams are appropriately prepared for the procedure. This includes review of anesthesia, airway management, and interventions, as well as developing a course of action for possible complications, incidental findings, and respiratory decompensation. Teaching should similarly occur before, during, and after clinical procedures.

Pre-operative briefing and post-operative debriefing have been shown to (1) promote a culture of safety within procedural fields, (2) increase goal-oriented and structured conversation between educators and learners, and (3) increase intra-operative verbal instruction, demonstration, observation of trainee performance, and delivery of constructive feedback. During pre-operative briefing, the learner should work with the educator to analyze past experiences, determine the current level of expertise and areas for improvement, and formulate intra-operative objectives. During post-operative debriefing, both parties should reflect upon the intra-operative encounter, as well as reinforcing learning points and correcting mistakes.[27]

PRACTICAL TRAINING FOR PEDIATRIC BRONCHOSCOPY – INTRA-OPERATIVE TEACHING

Given concerns for patient safety, as well as institutional pressures to increase clinical productivity and minimize the cost of OR utilization, surgical faculty need an efficient and effective approach to intra-operative teaching and evaluation. The Zwisch model, a system that defines four milestones of operative development, may be useful for advancing and assessing trainees in the bronchoscopy suite. According to this model, a trainee transitions from the "Show and Tell" to "Smart Help" to "Dumb Help" to "No Help" stages of intra-operative supervision. As they do so, their role evolves from observer to first assistant to primary surgeon requiring active assistance to primary surgeon requiring passive assistance. A standardized, instructional method such as this establishes transparent expectations and criteria for granting and earning autonomy in the OR. This can enhance OR learning environments by guiding both student preparation and faculty educational planning.[28]

Pediatric bronchoscopy cases are highly variable in complexity and acuity. Therefore, trainees should master routine diagnostic techniques before transitioning to more difficult interventional skills. Teachers should ensure that trainees see variety in patient acuity and diagnoses (see Table 10.3). For flexible bronchoscopy, this may also include the location of procedure (intensive care unit (ICU), procedure center, or operating room) as well as the mode of entry (nasal, endotracheal tube, or laryngeal mask airway) and the reasons to select the above.

A limitation to applying the Zwisch model to pediatric bronchoscopy teaching is that this technique has fewer opportunities for first assistant than other surgical procedures. However, a scope can easily be transitioned between individuals. Thus, a trainee can be allotted more time as the primary surgeon/proceduralist as they gradually earn autonomy. Additionally, in order to accurately monitor a trainee's progression, programs must develop formative and summative evaluation tools that are easily incorporated into faculty members' busy schedules.[28]

ACCREDITATION: TRAINING REQUIREMENTS AND COMPETENCY ASSESSMENT TOOLS

Cognitive aspects of pediatric bronchoscopy may be evaluated using multiple-choice or case-based questionnaires. These may be self-directed using available web-based curricula or in the form of validated in-service and board examinations.[9,10,21]

Historically, proficiency in a procedural skill has been measured quantitatively *via* minimum case numbers and/or qualitatively *via* evaluations from supervisors.[9–11,14,21] Pediatric Otolaryngology fellowships in the United States (US) range between one and two years. The Accreditation Council for Graduate Medical Education (ACGME) requires candidates to complete a minimum of 50 cases per year within the "Endoscopy with Intervention" domain. This includes laryngoscopy, bronchoscopy, and/or esophagoscopy with intervention. Similarly, a survey of pediatric pulmonary fellowship directors reported that the mean suggested number of flexible bronchoscopies for fellows to perform during fellowship was 50 procedures (Leong et al.[8]). The limitations of volume-based certification systems include arbitrarily defined thresholds based on expert opinion instead of scientific evidence and the lack of flexibility to accommodate individuals with different learning curves and rates of skill acquisition. Although evaluations allow for a more open-ended assessment of a trainee's performance, they do not provide timely feedback and can be influenced by recall and other innate biases.[9,10,21]

Given these limitations, multiple surgical disciplines are working to establish validated tools that would allow "skill acquisition and knowledge-based competency assessment for trainees".[21] One simple tool for the assessment of technical skill is hand motion. The number and size of hand motions is significantly inversely correlated with surgeon experience and surgical success.[29] In other words, individuals with the most experience use subtle and precise hand movements, whereas trainees use more, larger, and less-precise hand movements. Observation of hand movements can allow teachers to assess their learners and help learners strive toward technical expertise.

The Rigid Bronchoscopy Tool for Assessment of Skills and Competence (RIGID-TASC) is a research-validated instrument designed to measure technical and interpretive skills in rigid bronchoscopy, as well as stent placement and thermal interventional techniques. Outcome measurements for rigid bronchoscopy include (1) first-attempt passage of scope into the trachea in more than 90% of cases without significant periods of hypoxia, (2) injury to surrounding structures in less than 2% of cases, and (3) therapeutic results.[3,10,14] Additionally, checklists, such as the Oxford Non-Technical Skills (NOTECHS) 10-scale, Non-Technical Skills in Surgery (NOTSS) scale, and Anesthetists' Non-Technical Skills (ANTS) behavior assessment tool, have been used to evaluate non-technical skills during simulated airway emergencies.[30,31]

Although only validated for flexible bronchoscopy procedures in adults, the Ontario Bronchoscopy Assessment Tool (OBAT) can be used to help educators assess learning competency.[32] Voduc and colleagues used the OBAT to understand how many procedures were needed for trainees to reach competence in flexible bronchoscopy. Although the study sample was small in size, the authors reported a great variability from 10 to over 100 procedures needed for a trainee to score in the "competent" range.[33] Ongoing work is needed to determine the best way to assess competency during brief encounters between learners and attending clinicians.

CONTINUOUS PROFESSIONAL DEVELOPMENT

Continuous professional development initiatives help established providers update their proficiencies and grow as educators, as well as guiding new graduates as they transition into practice.[10] "Boot camps" use interactive didactic sessions and simulation exercises to take participants "from theory to practice".[10,14] Many programs also provide formal training in leadership and practice management. Components of practice management include, but are not limited to, billing and coding, reimbursement, insurance approval, professional liability, and quality improvement processes.

Bronchoscopy International has developed a "Train-the-Trainers" course[17] to help educators learn how to design student-centered curricula, deconstruct difficult topics, facilitate case-based discussion, lead interactive didactic sessions, provide constructive feedback, and use assessment tools. Though this course was designed for individuals teaching flexible bronchoscopy, its principles are also applicable for pediatric rigid bronchoscopy education.[9]

FUTURE OPPORTUNITIES

Many of the physical models available for airway education realistically depict supraglottic anatomy, making them strong training modalities for intubation. This is likely because intubation training spans multiple disciplines, including otolaryngology, anesthesiology, and emergency medicine. There exists a need for simulators that provide sufficiently detailed views of glottic, subglottic, tracheal, and bronchial anatomy. This gap is being addressed with advances in 3D-printing technology.

As image processing and digital reconstruction becomes more accessible, 3D printing may be used to design patient-specific pathologic models that providers can use to practice difficult navigation or complex interventional techniques. 3D printers can combine various polymers to mimic a broad spectrum of tissue and mechanical properties. Although the cost of printing varies according to design complexity and choice of materials, it has been estimated that most 3D rigid bronchoscopy models can be produced for less than $100. This is significantly lower than the cost of either low- or high-fidelity commercial physical simulators.[34]

For the average bronchoscopist, staying up to date on the most current technology can feel difficult. National societies, other organizations, or individual institutions need to help disseminate current information as technology changes.

CONCLUSION

Bronchoscopy is crucial for the evaluation and treatment of routine and emergency pediatric airway conditions. Novel instructional methods are providing interactive and safe opportunities to learn theoretical principles and develop practical skills for this technique. However, there is a need to standardize training requirements across pediatric pulmonology and otolaryngology programs, using measurable competency metrics as opposed to volume-based criteria. Continued optimization and validation of simulators, assessment tools, and student/faculty curricula will help improve and regulate pediatric bronchoscopy education.

TIPS FOR CLINICAL EDUCATION

1. Use open-ended questions and examples to assess your learner's current stage of knowledge.
2. Learning a procedural skill requires the compilation of medical knowledge, technical skills, and clinical practice.
3. A combination of novel didactics, low-fidelity and high-fidelity simulation, bedside, and intra-operative training should be used to teach (and learn) bronchoscopy.
4. Assessments of initial competency, as well as ongoing competency and maintenance of certification, should be incorporated into bronchoscopy practice.

REFERENCES

1. Pastis NJ, Nietert PJ, Silvestri GA. Variation in training for interventional pulmonary procedures among US pulmonary/critical care fellowships: A survey of fellowship directors. *Chest [Internet]*. 2005;127(5):1614–21. Available from: http://dx.doi.org/10.1378/chest.127.5.1614
2. Stather DR, Jarand J, Silvestri GA, Tremblay A. An evaluation of procedural training in Canadian respirology fellowship programs: Program directors' and fellows' perspectives. *Can Respir J*. 2009;16(2):55–9.
3. Mahmood K, Wahidi MM, Osann KE, Coles K, Shofer SL, Volker EE, et al. Development of a tool to assess basic competency in the performance of rigid bronchoscopy. *Ann Am Thorac Soc*. 2016;13(4):502–11.
4. Amin MR, Friedmann DR. Simulation-based training in advanced airway skills in an otolaryngology residency program. *Laryngoscope*. 2013;123(3):629–34.
5. Knox DB, Wong WW. Graduating fellows' procedural comfort level with pulmonary critical care procedures. *J Bronchol Interv Pulmonol*. 2019;26(4):231–6.
6. Hsiung GE, Schwab B, O'Brien EK, Gause CD, Hebal F, Barsness KA, et al. Preliminary evaluation of a novel rigid bronchoscopy simulator. *J Laparoendosc Adv Surg Tech*. 2017;27(7):737–43.
7. Shah RK, Patel A, Lander L, Choi SS. Management of foreign bodies obstructing the airway in children. *Arch Otolaryngol: Head Neck Surg*. 2010;136(4):373–9.
8. Leong AB, Green CG, Kurland G, Wood RE. A survey of training in pediatric flexible bronchoscopy. *Pediatr Pulmonol*. 2014;49(6):605–10.
9. Fielding DI, Maldonado F, Murgu S. Achieving competency in bronchoscopy: Challenges and opportunities. *Respirology*. 2014;19(4):472–82.
10. Corbetta L. Training to competence in interventional pulmonology. *Panminerva Med*. 2019;61(3):201–2.
11. Hunyady A, Polaner D. Pediatric airway management education and training. *Paediatr Anaesth*. 2020;30(3):362–70.
12. Langlois J, Wells GA, Lecourtois M, Bergeron G, Yetisir E, Martin M. Spatial abilities of medical graduates and choice of residency programs. *Anat Sci Educ*. 2015;8(2):111–9.
13. Jabbour N, Reihsen T, Sweet RM, Sidman JD. Psychomotor skills training in pediatric airway endoscopy simulation. *Otolaryngol: Head Neck Surg*. 2011;145(1):43–50.
14. Galluccio G, Tramaglino LM, Marchese R, Bandelli GP, Vigliar Olo R, Corbetta L. Competence in operative bronchoscopy. *Panminerva Med*. 2019;61(3):298–325.

15. Harless J, Ramaiah R, Bhananker SM. Symposium: Critical airway management pediatric airway management. *Int J Crit Illn Inj Sci*. 2014;4(1):65–70.

16. Raj D, Luginbuehl I. Managing the difficult airway in the syndromic child. *Contin Educ Anaesthesia, Crit Care Pain*. 2015;15(1):7–13.

17. Bronchoscopy International [Internet]. Available from: https://bronchoscopy.org/essential -bronchoscopist

18. Kennedy CC, Maldonado F, Cook DA. Simulation-based bronchoscopy training: Systematic review and meta-analysis. *Chest*. 2013;144(1):183–92.

19. Boyd AD. Chevalier Jackson: The father of American bronchoesophagoscopy. *Ann Thorac Surg [Internet]*. 1994;57(2):502–5. Available from: http://dx.doi.org/10.1016/0003-4975(94)91037-5

20. Javia L, Deutsch ES. A systematic review of simulators in otolaryngology. *Otolaryngol: Head Neck Surg*. 2012;147(6):999–1011.

21. Ernst A, Wahidi MM, Read CA, Buckley JD, Addrizzo-Harris DJ, Shah PL, et al. Adult bronchoscopy training: Current state and suggestions for the future: CHEST expert panel report. *Chest [Internet]*. 2015;148(2):321–32. Available from: http://dx.doi.org/10.1378/chest.14-0678

22. Ram B, Oluwole M, Blair RL, Mountain R, Dunkley P, White PS. Surgical simulation: An animal tissue model for training in therapeutic and diagnostic bronchoscopy. *J Laryngol Otol*. 1999;113(2):149–51.

23. Al-Ramahi J, Luo H, Fang R, Chou A, Jiang J, Kille T. Development of an innovative 3D printed rigid bronchoscopy training model. *Ann Otol Rhinol Laryngol*. 2016;125(12):965–9.

24. Deboer EM, Wagner J, Kroehl ME, Albietz J, Shandas R, Deterding RR, et al. Three-dimensional printed pediatric airway model improves novice learners' flexible bronchoscopy skills with minimal direct teaching from faculty. *Simul Healthc*. 2018;13(4):284–8.

25. Deutsch ES, Dixit D, Curry J, Malloy K, Christenson T, Robinson B, et al. Management of aerodigestive tract foreign bodies: Innovative teaching concepts. *Ann Otol Rhinol Laryngol*. 2007;116(5):319–23.

26. Griffin GR, Hoesli R, Thorne MC. Validity and efficacy of a pediatric airway foreign body training course in resident education. *Ann Otol Rhinol Laryngol*. 2011;120(10):635–40.

27. Roberts NK, Williams RG, Kim MJ, Dunnington GL. The briefing, intraoperative teaching, debriefing model for teaching in the operating room. *J Am Coll Surg [Internet]*. 2009;208(2):299–303. Available from: http://dx.doi.org/10.1016/j.jamcollsurg.2008.10.024

28. Darosa DA, Zwischenberger JB, Meyerson SL, George BC, Teitelbaum EN, Soper NJ, et al. A theory-based model for teaching and assessing residents in the operating room. *J Surg Educ [Internet]*. 2013;70(1):24–30. Available from: http://dx.doi.org/10.1016/j.jsurg.2012.07.007

29. Datta V, Chang A, Mackay S, Darzi A. The relationship between motion analysis and surgical technical assessments. *Am J Surg*. 2002;184(1):70–3.

30. Mishra A, Catchpole K, Mcculloch P. The Oxford NOTECHS system: Reliability and validity of a tool for measuring teamwork behaviour In the operating theatre. *Qual Saf Heal Care*. 2009;18(2):104–8.

31. Wu KY, Kim S, Fung K, Roth K. Assessing nontechnical skills in otolaryngology emergencies through simulation-based training. *Laryngoscope*. 2018;128(10):2301–6.

32. Voduc N, Dudek N, Parker CM, Sharma KB, Wood TJ. Development and validation of a bronchoscopy competence assessment tool in a clinical setting. *Ann Am Thorac Soc*. 2016;13(4):495–501.

33. Voduc N, Adamson R, Kashgari A, Fenton M, Porhownick N, Wojnar M, et al. Development of learning curves for bronchoscopy: Results of a multicenter study of pulmonary trainees. *Chest [Internet]*. 2020;158(6):2485–92. Available from: http://dx.doi.org/10.1016/j.chest.2020.06.046

34. Leong TL, Li J. 3D printed airway simulators: Adding a dimension to bronchoscopy training. *Respirology*. 2020;25(11):1126–8.

11

Airway management and anesthetic considerations

MELISSA BROOKS PETERSON, PELTON PHINIZY, AND JEREMY D. PRAGER

INTRODUCTION

Anesthesia and airway management for pediatric bronchoscopy is dynamic, collaborative, and requires clinical expertise and familiarity with equipment in order for it to be performed safely and successfully. Location, timing, goals of the procedure, clinical condition of the patient, and a wide variety of options for airway and anesthetic management strategies are the most important factors to consider when performing pediatric bronchoscopy. Multidisciplinary decision making pre-, intra-, and post-procedure is critical to ensuring a safe, efficient, and useful procedure, whether it is diagnostic or therapeutic. In-depth knowledge of airway equipment and adjuncts, as well as open communication, are the most important factors for successful completion of both routine and high-risk pediatric bronchoscopy.

LOCATION – BEDSIDE/INTENSIVE CARE UNIT *VERSUS* OPERATING ROOM/ENDOSCOPY SUITE

The choice of where to perform pediatric bronchoscopy depends on a number of factors and must be driven primarily by the predicted ability to answer the clinical question or achieve the desired intervention in the safest, most efficient manner.

- The patient's clinical condition is the most important determinant of the location for pediatric bronchoscopy. The clinical features that should be considered include the patient's current airway status (e.g., natural airway, non-invasive ventilation, mechanical ventilation with intubation), need for supplemental oxygen, level of oxygen requirement, need for inhaled humidified air, need for inhaled nitric oxide, respiratory rate, work of breathing at baseline, work of breathing under duress or stress, and

DOI: 10.1201/9781003106234-11

other vital signs including oxyhemoglobin saturation, heart rate, temperature, and cardiac rhythm. An additional consideration is the presence, absence, and number of continuous medication infusions the patient requires and if those can be safely paused or continued during transport. Transporting a patient from their hospital location may increase risk because it requires altering or even disconnecting airway and physiologic support. The determination of whether it is clinically appropriate to move a patient should be determined in a multidisciplinary fashion with anesthesiologists, proceduralists (pulmonologists and/or otolaryngologists), as well as representation from the patient's primary team and nursing staff. If a patient cannot be safely transported due to severe illness or the inability to continue supportive and life-sustaining measures during transport, performing the procedure in the intensive care unit (ICU) may be the only option. In these circumstances, limitations of the procedure itself should be recognized, including more limited space and equipment, as well as less-experienced personnel. Efforts to minimize these limitations may be required.

- Equipment factors are also a vital consideration in determining where to perform pediatric bronchoscopy. These factors include immediate equipment availability and equipment expertise. Having immediate access to comprehensive airway equipment is critical to the pulmonologist, otolaryngologist, and anesthesiologist being able to safely and successfully perform the procedure. Having personnel on hand who are familiar with equipment for these fields, where the equipment is located, and how to assemble and utilize it, is a part of this determinant. The tools and personnel are most often located in an operating room (OR) or comparable procedure room. Critical equipment includes multiple types of laryngoscope blades, multiple types of scopes (both rigid and flexible), high-definition cameras, screens and recording devices, and monitoring capabilities.

- Optimal staffing is another vital determinant in the ideal location for pediatric bronchoscopy. The presence of a pediatric anesthesiologist, proceduralist (pediatric pulmonologist and/or otolaryngologist), and support staff is a key consideration. Pediatric anesthesiologists have the most familiarity with sedation and/or general anesthesia for performing optimal pediatric bronchoscopy, transporting critical patients, the presence of comprehensive monitoring, the precise titration of medications for a static and dynamic airway examination, and familiarity with the dynamic nature of the procedure itself, procedural complications and their management. Operating room and post-anesthesia care unit nursing staff are the most familiar with recovering pediatric bronchoscopy patients and the challenges they can present. For a patient who can tolerate being safely transported to the OR, it is preferable to perform pediatric bronchoscopy in the OR where equipment availability, equipment familiarity and expertise, consultant expertise, and staffing are ideal. In cases in which a patient is too critically ill to transport (e.g., extracorporeal membrane oxygenation [ECMO]) or in which the therapeutic goal is discrete and the anticipated procedure very short (e.g., bronchoscopy in a stable, intubated patient for suctioning of a presumed mucus plug), it is reasonable to perform at the bedside.

AIRWAY SECUREMENT

The choice of airway management for pediatric bronchoscopy is highly nuanced. Each airway device has specific benefits and limitations that require consideration. Some considerations include procedure-specific goals and patient-specific factors. Pediatric bronchoscopy can be performed *via* an endotracheal tube (ETT), a tracheostomy tube, a supraglottic device, or nasally or orally *via* a natural airway.

- Bronchoscopy *via* ETT is a reasonable option for patients who require evaluation of the lower trachea, bronchus, and/or bronchioles. It is also a useful airway device if the goals of the procedure are to perform bronchoalveolar lavage for diagnostic or therapeutic purposes, as the ETT provides a straight conduit to the lower airways as well as a seal *via* an inflated ETT cuff to protect the airway, if desired. A double-lumen ETT can also be used for whole lung lavage, though in pediatric patients a double-lumen ETT can be difficult to place due to the large external diameter of the device. In the case of size limitation, a single-lumen tube advanced into either mainstem bronchus may be preferred. ETT for bronchoscopy can be quite useful for diagnostic or therapeutic interventions in patients who are very ill and/or have tenuous oxygenation, who require the support of positive-pressure ventilation during general anesthesia, or who may otherwise decompensate without the support of mechanical ventilation and delivery of supplemental oxygen during the procedure. Limitations of performing bronchoscopy *via* ETT include the size of equipment; the internal diameter of the ETT may limit the size of a pediatric flexible bronchoscope that can be passed without obstructing oxygenation and ventilation and maneuvered without damaging the scope itself. Additionally, introducing a flexible bronchoscope into the lumen of the ETT creates obstruction, which could potentially lead to dynamic hyperinflation and auto-positive end-expiratory pressure (PEEP).[1,2] Additionally, the ETT obscures the oropharynx, pharynx, larynx, and upper trachea, so it is less ideal if these anatomic regions are of interest to the pediatric pulmonologist or otolaryngologist. In addition, the tube's presence in the trachea changes the dynamic evaluation of this portion of the airway. Although many modes of ventilation can be employed during flexible bronchoscopy *via* ETT, usually some degree of positive-pressure ventilation is needed to overcome the resistance of the ETT and obstruction by a flexible scope so that adequate oxygenation and ventilation can be achieved during the procedure. These factors limit the evaluation of tracheobronchomalacia.

- Pediatric bronchoscopy can also be performed *via* a tracheostomy tube. Utilizing this type of airway device depends again on the clinical question to be answered and the goals of the procedure. This also requires precise communication between the anesthesiology and surgical teams pre-induction. The native tracheostomy device can be left in place, recognizing that, if the device has an air leak around it, this may pose a challenge for effective anesthesia gas exchange, oxygenation and/or ventilation, and supplemental oxygen delivery. If the leak is too large to maintain the patient's physiology, exchanging the device for a larger or cuffed device or endotracheal tube may be the best option. Bronchoscopy can also be performed through the tracheal stoma (removing the tracheal tube entirely) for improved examination of the stomal site or through the nasal or oral cavity in a patient with a tracheostomy, depending on the anatomic areas of interest. In most cases, it is ideal to keep these patients spontaneously breathing throughout the procedure to facilitate requested changes in airway management, anesthesia gas, and oxygen delivery and to ensure a safe, effective, and efficient procedure. If needed to support oxygenation or ventilation, assisted mechanical ventilation settings can be employed.

- Bronchoscopy can be performed *via* a supraglottic airway (SGA), (e.g., laryngeal mask airways [LMA], Teleflex, Wayne, PA, USA). An SGA is placed transorally and bypasses the oropharynx, providing access to the larynx, subglottis, trachea, and distal airways. It forms a seal in the hypopharynx, allowing for effective delivery of oxygen and anesthesia gas, and facilitates monitoring of oxygenation, ventilation, and gas exchange; usually an SGA can seal up to a pressure of between 10 and 20 cm H_2O.[3,4] This is usually adequate for pediatric lungs with normal compliance but can be a limiting step for patients with poor lung compliance, higher oxygen requirements, or other pathology. For a short, efficient bronchoscopy procedure, an SGA is a reasonable method of providing adequate oxygenation and ventilation (in a spontaneous or controlled mode of ventilation) while simultaneously giving the bronchoscopist access to the larynx, glottic opening, upper trachea, and the remainder of the distal airways. Limitations of using an SGA for pediatric bronchoscopy include limited generation of positive pressure, limiting the view of the oropharynx, hypopharynx, and supraglottic larynx, and changing the native position of the larynx with a properly seated SGA (a properly seated SGA moves the larynx posterior and caudad, and tilts the laryngeal inlet posteriorly). Fiber-optic intubation via a SGA is described in Chapter 6.

- Pediatric bronchoscopy *via* a natural airway may offer the most accurate assessment of a patient's airway anatomy from nasopharynx or oropharynx to the distal airway. The bronchoscopist may assess the patient's entire airway under spontaneously breathing conditions, *via* negative inspiratory pressure, which more closely resembles natural breathing, and in the absence of devices that alter airway geometry (ETT, SGA). This is an ideal method to assess tracheobronchomalacia.[5] The challenges of performing bronchoscopy *via* the natural airway include patient selection (considering patient factors that may prevent safe bronchoscopy), goals of the procedure (considering the clinical question to be answered or therapeutic goals and choosing an appropriate airway management strategy), and performing the procedure itself without hypoxemia, hypercarbia, or other physiologic decompensation. Additionally, with a natural airway, there is the challenge of increased stimulation of passage of a scope across the nasopharynx or oropharynx, which requires teamwork and communication so that the patient remains within a plane of anesthesia that is deep enough to tolerate the procedural stimulation, but light enough that the patient can maintain spontaneous ventilation, adequate oxygenation, and ventilation, and achieve ideal conditions for a goal-directed examination by the bronchoscopist.

- Standard monitors must be used for the duration of the procedure, including gas sample analysis (for the fraction of inspired oxygen [FiO_2] and CO_2), regardless of the mode of ventilation employed, keeping in mind that the absolute values may change depending on the mode of ventilation, the degree of the leak, and the patient's respiratory status. This can be interpreted and adjusted by the pediatric anesthesiologist, who is familiar with the limitations of gas sample analysis during open airway procedures.

- During bronchoscopy with a natural airway, there are a number of ways to supply supplemental oxygen and/or assist ventilation. It is routine to deliver supplemental oxygen *via* the bronchoscope channel itself, recognizing the small but real risk of too much flow and the risk of pneumothorax or hyperinflation.[6,7] The same channel is also used for suctioning, so it may not be reliable for continuous delivery. As seen in **Figure 11.1A–C**, supplemental oxygen can also be delivered by blow-by *via* mask (**11.1A**), blow-by *via* circuit placed in the oral cavity (**11.1B**), or by anesthesia face mask (**11.1C**). A modified nasal trumpet is another highly effective way to deliver supplemental oxygen and obtain gas sample analysis during bronchoscopy *via* the natural airway (**Figure 11.2A–C**). A modified nasal trumpet inserted into the naris allows the delivery of oxygen and gas sample analysis while preserving the natural anatomy and respiratory physiology of the contralateral naris, oral, pharyngeal, laryngeal, and tracheobronchial cavities. Other maneuvers that help facilitate flexible bronchoscopy include the extension of the head (to more properly align the nasal, oropharyngeal, and tracheal planes) or jaw thrust (to relieve obstruction and improve access to the laryngeal inlet with the flexible bronchoscope).

- It is also possible to deliver positive-pressure breaths or continuous positive airway pressure by face mask *during* a flexible bronchoscopy. This requires a true "shared airway" between the pediatric anesthesiologist and pediatric pulmonologist/otolaryngologist. The flexible scope can be left in place, rested slightly caudad and laterally against the patient's cheek, and the anesthesia face mask with attached circuit placed over the flexible scope (**Video 11.1, Video 11.2, Figure 11.3**). It is frequently possible to achieve a mask seal and deliver supplemental oxygen, reverse atelectasis by applying continuous positive airway pressure (CPAP) or PEEP by mask and improve oxygenation and ventilatory parameters during the bronchoscopy in parallel with the procedure. The most important role of this technique is to support oxygenation and ventilation *without* having to abort or interrupt the procedure. This method is particularly useful for patients who desaturate quickly due to poor pulmonary reserve or due to

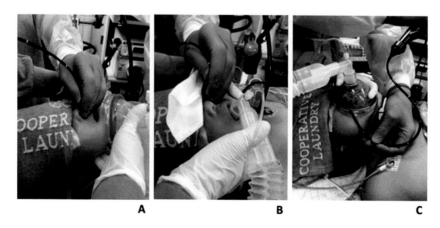

A   **B**   **C**

Figure 11.1 There are several vehicles by which to deliver supplemental oxygen during bronchoscopy: blow-by *via* mask (A), blow-by *via* circuit placed in the oral cavity (B), or by anesthesia face mask (C).

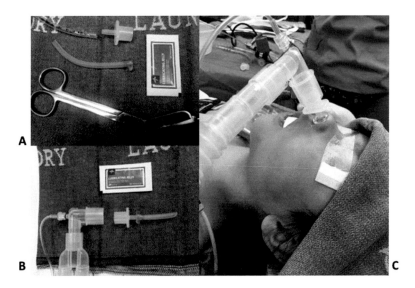

Figure 11.2 (A–C) A modified nasal trumpet is used to deliver supplemental oxygen and obtain gas sample analysis during bronchoscopy *via* a natural airway.

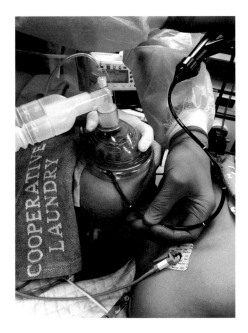

Figure 11.3 A flexible bronchoscope is rested against the patient's cheek, while a face mask with the attached circuit is placed over the flexible scope.

pulmonary disease, patients at the extremes of age who have reduced functional residual capacity (FRC) and reduced closing capacity, or procedures that take a longer time than usual and therefore predispose to atelectasis and desaturation.

Video 11.1 A flexible bronchoscope is rested against the patient's cheek and an anesthesia face mask is used.

In summary, there is an armamentarium of airway maneuvers, devices, and methods to deliver supplemental oxygen and improve ventilation during pediatric bronchoscopy. It is the shared responsibility of the pediatric anesthesiologist, pulmonologist, and otolaryngologist to employ the appropriate maneuvers to facilitate a safe, efficient, and goal-directed bronchoscopy, and to communicate before, during, and after the procedure for the best possible patient outcome. It is frequently the case that the goals of the procedure require a native or natural anatomic airway, and the patient's physiology during the procedure necessitates supportive maneuvers. Sometimes, the patient will benefit from one or more methods of airway support or control during a bronchoscopy (e.g., starting with a natural airway for upper airway evaluation, and switching to an SGA or ETT to add the ability to apply supportive ventilation and oxygenation). Use of the best strategy for airway management during bronchoscopy (with a single or multiple approaches) is a dynamic, collaborative effort whereby communication, flexibility, and adjustments to the plan by the entire procedural team should become routine.

MEDICATIONS FOR PEDIATRIC BRONCHOSCOPY

Medications used for pediatric bronchoscopy include sedative/hypnotics, opioids, anesthetic gases, intravenous anesthetics, local anesthetic, and others. These medications can be used pre-, intra-, and post-operatively to optimize the anesthesia for both patient tolerance and successful procedural outcomes.

- Pre-operatively, it is occasionally appropriate to premedicate a child who will have a difficult time separating from parents or caregivers for the induction of anesthesia. In cases where distraction techniques, parental presence, environmental controls, and/or non-pharmacologic relaxation techniques are not effective, sedatives can be administered to decrease pre-procedural anxiety.[8] The most common pre-procedural medications include oral midazolam (usually 0.5 mg/kg bodyweight up to 20 mg maximum) or intranasal dexmedetomidine (0.5–1 mcg/kg) and, less commonly, intranasal midazolam. Oral or intranasal midazolam has the benefit of rapid-onset sedation and anxiolysis but causes decreased respiratory drive especially in combination with other anesthetic or analgesic medications. Dexmedetomidine provides sedation without respiratory depression but has a longer onset. Both medications have a sedative effect for 2–6 hours after the procedure, so recovery conditions and disposition of the patient should be considered before administration.
- Anesthetic medications used to achieve and maintain general anesthesia during pediatric bronchoscopy include intravenous sedative/hypnotics[9] and anesthetic gases.[10] All sedative/hypnotic or anesthetic medications have a variety of dose-dependent side effects and a spectrum of desired clinical effects depending on the timing, route, and dose administered. Although this is beyond the scope of this chapter, it is a routine practice of all anesthesiologists to manage the nuances of medication for pediatric bronchoscopy. All classes and types of sedative/hypnotics can be used alone, in combination, or omitted from the anesthetic plan entirely, depending on a variety of patient and procedural considerations.
  - Propofol is a gamma-aminobutyric acid type A receptor agonist (GABA-ergic), a sedative/hypnotic, and is the most common intravenous general anesthetic medication used for pediatric bronchoscopy. It is very short acting and can be carefully titrated for a variety of effects ranging from sedation to general anesthesia with or without apnea. There is no one dose that is effective for any single patient, procedure, or clinical effect, but, when correctly titrated for the desired clinical effect and in consideration of patient and procedural factors, propofol is a highly useful and safe medication.[9]
  - Other sedative/hypnotics or general anesthetics include etomidate, which is usually reserved for induction of anesthesia in hemodynamically unstable patients, and ketamine, which provides

dose-dependent dissociation from painful stimuli and can also induce general anesthesia. One significant downside highly relevant to pediatric bronchoscopy is that ketamine causes significant secretion production throughout the upper and lower airways and is therefore not an optimal anesthetic agent for many pediatric bronchoscopy procedures.[9]

- Inhaled fluorinated anesthetic gases ("-fluranes") can also be used. Most commonly, sevoflurane is used for inhaled induction of anesthesia, given that it is the least noxious of the anesthetic gases (for tolerance of inhaled induction), and has very low solubility, which results in a rapid onset and offset.[10]

- Opioids are another useful class of medication that can be administered during pediatric bronchoscopy.[11] Most commonly, a short-acting and potent opioid such as fentanyl is utilized to treat pain and stimulation from the bronchoscopy itself and has the benefit of some pain control in the post-anesthesia care unit. Other benefits of fentanyl are that it is titratable and predictable in its pharmacologic effects. Regardless of the opioid administered, it is critical to choose a dose and timing of administration that will preserve spontaneous ventilation. A dose that is too large or administered at the wrong time may result in apnea that may prevent the achievement of a particular procedure's goals and may cause desaturation and/or hemodynamic instability. Whereas dose-dependent respiratory depression is the downside of using any opioid during bronchoscopy, its use may facilitate a balanced anesthetic technique and minimize the effects of the painful or stimulating portions of the bronchoscopy.

- Local or topical anesthesia is commonly used.[12] Administration of atomized or topical lidocaine (ranging from 1% to 4%) to the larynx prior to bronchoscopy can reduce the effects of surgical stimulation and also reduce the risk of laryngospasm by decreasing the sensitivity of the vocal cords during the invasive procedure. Lidocaine may be used topically on the carina and lower airways to reduce the cough reflex associated with stimulating the trachea with the bronchoscope. Lidocaine may also be administered intravenously (1–2 mg/kg) to reduce the cough response to tracheal, carinal, or lower airway stimulation. Regardless of the mode of delivery of local anesthetics, it is critical for the pediatric anesthesiologist, pulmonologist, and otolaryngologist to communicate about the total dosage of all local anesthetics for the entire procedure prior to any administration to avoid putting the patient at risk of systemic toxicity due to overdose. The typical upper limits of lidocaine are 3 mg/kg (plain) and 5 mg/kg (with epinephrine).

- Topical vasoconstrictors (e.g., intranasal oxymetazoline) are commonly used in the nares prior to bronchoscopy to decongest the nasal mucosa and reduce the risk of traumatic epistaxis. There are concerns regarding the systemic effects of these medications, and their judicious, limited use is recommended.[13,14] Steroids are administered during bronchoscopy as a treatment for potential airway edema in response to the procedure. The most commonly selected steroid is dexamethasone (0.5 mg/kg intravenous to a maximum of 8–12 mg), which reduces pain post-procedure and also decreases the occurrence of postoperative nausea and vomiting. The final class of medication that is used, albeit rarely, in bronchoscopy are neuromuscular blocking agents (paralytics). These agents should be used on a case-by-case basis, where a controlled mode of ventilation with paralysis is the only viable option for performing the procedure. Communication before the procedure, including an algorithmic approach to ventilation in the event of apnea, is required.

COMPLICATIONS DURING PEDIATRIC BRONCHOSCOPY

The most common complications during pediatric bronchoscopy include agitation during the procedure or intolerance of inhaled induction, hypoxemia, hypercapnia, laryngospasm, and bronchospasm. Although all of these complications are usually avoidable and/or treatable when they do occur, it is important to be prepared to respond to each of these. The procedural needs and method of bronchoscopy, paired with the anesthetic management of bronchoscopy, can precipitate these complications but can also be integral to avoiding the same complications altogether. This is one of the major benefits of performing pediatric bronchoscopy in the most controlled setting possible (the operating room or procedural center), so that, if these complications do arise, the patient is cared for by the optimal team in the most controlled environment.

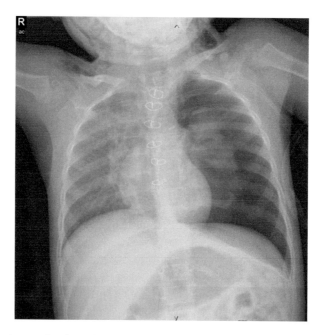

Figure 11.4 Pneumothorax after bronchoscopy. The risk of major complications is higher in patients with serious or life-threatening comorbidities, patients at the extremes of age (e.g., prematurity), and those with congenital cardiac disease and/or pulmonary hypertension as well as children undergoing lung biopsy.

It is important to remember that some of these complications will present in the recovery unit. Patients with cough, stridor, hypoxemia, and a new supplemental oxygen requirement may be experiencing residual mild problems from the procedure and may need more observation time. They may also be experiencing something more significant (**Figure 11.4**).

Serious complications, like pneumothorax, cardiac arrest, and the need for cardiopulmonary resuscitation, are usually precipitated by airway trauma (including barotrauma), airway compromise, or a respiratory complication (e.g., bradycardic arrest due to hypoxemia). The risk of major complications is higher in patients with serious or life-threatening co-morbidities, patients at the extremes of age (e.g., prematurity), and those with congenital cardiac disease and/or pulmonary hypertension. The ability of a multidisciplinary pediatric bronchoscopy team to respond quickly and appropriately to any complication is critical to ensuring the safety and efficacy of a pediatric bronchoscopy.

CONCLUSION

Pediatric bronchoscopy requires an experienced, communicative, and flexible team. Each individual on the team possesses various options for a procedural methodology that can be tailored to the patient and the information needed from this particular bronchoscopy. This is as true of the anesthesia provider as it is of the bronchoscopist. Part of this team discussion involves choosing the ideal setting for the procedure. While there is no "best" way to perform pediatric bronchoscopy, it is best practice for all team members to have familiarity with the patient as well as a working knowledge of the equipment and anesthetic options. It is common for the pediatric otolaryngologist, pulmonologist, and anesthesiologist to need to change plans in real-time, based on the patient's response to anesthesia, findings during the bronchoscopy, and the need for both static and dynamic airway evaluations. It is expected that patients will have some degree of hypoxemia and hypercarbia during bronchoscopy, and both the occurrence and effect of these physiologic derangements can be minimized (and therefore complications avoided) by having an efficient setup, communicative and nimble bronchoscopy team, and a plan set ahead of time for any complications that may arise.

TIPS FOR CLINICAL PRACTICE

- Location
  - Choose the OR or endoscopy/procedural suite if at all possible. Provided that the patient can be safely transported to the procedural location, the entire team will be most familiar with this setting, have the best access to all of the necessary equipment, and be prepared to respond appropriately to an emergency or complication.
  - Performing pediatric bronchoscopy in an OR or a dedicated procedural space also ensures the presence of personnel familiar with bronchoscopy, bronchoscopy equipment, and complications arising during the procedure.
- Airway management during pediatric bronchoscopy is dynamic and comprehensive and requires superb communication. Be sure to plan to have a full complement of airway equipment, and otolaryngologist, anesthesiologist, and procedural support staff available; this will depend on the patient as well as the goals of the procedure itself (therapeutic, diagnostic, or both) and should be planned ahead of time.
  - Use a natural airway, if possible (patient not intubated).
  - Use a supraglottic airway, if needed.
  - Standard monitoring needs can be met or approximated.
  - Oxygenation and ventilation can be assisted in a variety of methods, though these efforts can change the geometry of the airway.
- Medications
  - Maintain spontaneous ventilation if at all possible.
  - Consider supportive modes of ventilation and/or intermittent re-recruitment or PEEP maneuvers to maintain physiologic stability of the patient. All airway maneuvers require communication and teamwork.
  - Topical lidocaine to the larynx, intravenous dexamethasone, propofol, and short-acting opioids work well for most children.
- Complications
  - Anticipate and plan for complications or difficulties at each step. It is best to discuss as a team how each of these issues would be handled and to work with a team that is familiar and comfortable with pediatric bronchoscopy.
  - Serious complications are rare.

REFERENCES

1. Hsia D, DiBlasi RM, Richardson P, Crotwell D, Debley J, Carter E. The effects of flexible bronchoscopy on mechanical ventilation in a pediatric lung model. *Chest.* 2009;135(1):33–40.
2. Lawson RW, Peters JI, Shelledy DC. Effects of fiberoptic bronchoscopy during mechanical ventilation in a lung model. *Chest.* 2000;118(3):824–831.
3. R H. Airway Management. In: Davis PJ, Cladis FP, eds. *Smith's Anesthesia for Infants and Children.* 9th ed. Philadelphia, PA: Elsevier; 2017:349–369.
4. Ramesh S, Jayanthi R. Supraglottic airway devices in children. *Indian J Anaesth.* 2011;55(5):476–482.
5. Wallis C, Alexopoulou E, Anton-Pacheco JL, et al. ERS statement on tracheomalacia and bronchomalacia in children. *Eur Respir J.* 2019;54(3).
6. Chan IA, Gamble JJ. Tension pneumothorax during flexible bronchoscopy in a nonintubated infant. *Paediatr Anaesth.* 2016;26(4):452–454.
7. Muthu V, Sehgal IS, Prasad KT, Agarwal R. Iatrogenic pneumothorax following vigorous suctioning of mucus plug during flexible bronchoscopy. *BMJ Case Rep.* 2019;12(10).
8. Cravero JP, RR. Sedation. In: Davis PJ, Cladis FP, eds. *Anesthesia for Infants and Children.* 9th ed. Philadelphia, PA: Elsevier; 2017:1055–1069.

9. Blasiole B, DP. Intravenous agents. In: Davis PJ, Cladis FP, eds. *Smith's Anesthesia for Infants and Children*. 9th ed. Philadelphia, PA: Elsevier; 2017:186–199.

10. Frawley G, DA. Inhaled agents. In: Davis PJ, Cladis FP, eds. *Smith's Anesthesia for Infants and Children*. 9th ed. Philadelphia, PA: Elsevier; 2017:200–213.

11. Pian PMT, GJ, Davis PJ. Opioids. In: Davis PJ, Cladis FP, ed. *Smith's Anesthesia for Infants and Children*. 9th ed. Philadelphia, PA: Elsevier; 2017:219–238.

12. Bosenberg A. Local anesthetic agents. In: Davis PJ, Cladis FP, eds. *Smith's Anesthesia for Infants and Children*. 9th ed. Philadelphia, PA: Elsevier; 2017:214–218.

13. Cartabuke R, Tobias JD, Jatana KR, et al. Topical nasal decongestant oxymetazoline: safety considerations for perioperative pediatric use. 2021;148(5). doi:10.1542/peds.2021-054271.

14. Latham GJ, Jardine DS. Oxymetazoline and hypertensive crisis in a child: can we prevent it? *Paediatr Anaesth*. 2013;23(10):952–956.

Index

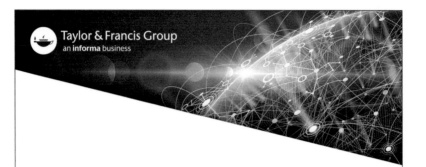